MANAGING A CARE HOME

An aide-memoire for nurses and care staff

Adrian M Ashurst, RGN, DMS

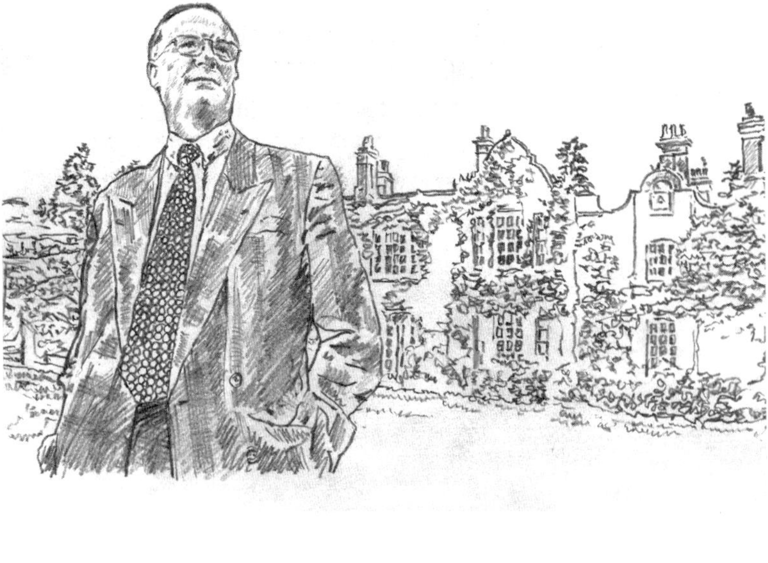

MANAGING A CARE HOME

An aide-memoire for nurses and care staff

Adrian M Ashurst, RGN, DMS

QUAY BOOKS
A division of MA Healthcare Ltd

Quay Books Division, MA Healthcare Ltd, St Jude's Church,
Dulwich Road, London SE24 0PB

British Library Cataloguing-in-Publication Data
A catalogue record is available for this book

ISBN-10 1 85642 231 3
ISBN-13 978 1 85642 231 4

Printed in Malta by Gutenberg Press, Gudja Road, Tarxien
PLA19, Malta

CONTENTS

FOREWORD

I am very pleased to have been asked to write the foreword for Adrian's new book. As chief executive of NHP Plc, responsible for owning or managing some three hundred and sixty care homes throughout the country, I was very interested in providing our care home managers and regional managers with sensible, common sense training materials which took advantage of the many years of collective experience that exists in our independent care sector.

Adrian's first 'how to' book entitled 'Positive Customer care – an aide- memoire' became a standard work for us in the process of training our staff. Whether from a nursing background or not, staff need to become focused on all aspects of customer care. It offered readers a real insight into the day-to-day issues which managers face while running a care home. This was particularly valuable coming from the viewpoint of a seasoned professional with over 35 years' experience of nursing and managing in both the NHS and the independent care sector.

This, his second book, is even better than the first and is filled with Adrian's own enthusiasm and knowledge of the care industry. Reflecting upon his personal anecdotes, Adrian provides the reader with a rare insight into the reality of care home management.

Having worked with Adrian at NHP's Highfield Care, I know how much it means to him to be able to share his vast experience and knowledge with those who are beginning, or even thinking of beginning, a career in care home management.

I hope you find 'Managing a Care Home' as useful as we at NHP found Adrian's first book. I would like to extend my best wishes to him for his future career in managing and developing those people who share in the important and rewarding task of caring for vulnerable people and their families.

Bill Colvin, Chairman of Southern Cross

For Sue, Brittany and Reece

Without the three of you this book would never have been completed. You inspire me to write every day and I appreciate what a wonderful nursing career I have and how much more there is to come in the future, God willing.

With all my love and thanks

Adrian

ACKNOWLEGEMENTS

Thanks to my children, Brittany and Reece for their patience and love.

A special thanks to Sue Naylor for her continuous encouragement, support and inspiration.

Thanks to my parents and to Stephen, an international artist who drew the illustration on the inside verso of this book, Carole and Paul, my sister and brothers, for their love.

I would also like to express my sincere thanks to those special people who have worked alongside me over many years, both in the National Health Service and the independent healthcare sector. Alan, Frank, Beryl, Graham, Maggie, Janet, John, Karen and not forgetting Anne Bailey, who have all shared the many exciting challenges, trials and tribulations associated with the management of care homes.

These experiences have given me the opportunity to write this book, which will try to capture the true essence of care management. Without these people's vast knowledge this book would have been much more difficult to complete.

Thanks to my colleagues at Nursing and Residential Care and Quay Books, Highbank, Robinia, Highfield (NHP) Craegmoor, Hallmark and Cambian Healthcare. Thanks also to Martin Conroy and all my colleagues at MCCM and Cambian Healthcare for their encouragement.

Adrian M Ashurst

INTRODUCTION

This book has been written to assist new care home managers, who are often faced with many diverse challenges upon their appointment.

I am going to reflect and share practical advice, based on my personal experiences in senior management gained over sixteen years overseeing many nursing and residential homes throughout the United Kingdom.

Today care home managers require an ability to be able to control both the business and care elements in order to manage a successful care home. At the same time, they need to facilitate the staff team to develop a centre of excellence and ensure that individuals receive high quality care and maximise their independence.

Many care home managers in the past have worked their way up through the ranks, but have never received any business management training.

Sole proprietors often denied the old-fashioned matrons any access to their business plans and budgets. Matrons only had to concern themselves with the clinical outcomes of their individual residents, with little or no responsibility for marketing and the financial aspects of managing the care business. This remains anecdotal evidence and it is easy to see why little was written about this period of time. Matrons would often have been afraid to speak out in public about their position within the care home.

To understand how the care home manager's role has evolved over the years, the background to the development of care homes requires a brief explanation.

Caring for older people has changed beyond recognition during the last three decades. As a student nurse in the early 1970s I remember clearly the Nightingale style wards in long-stay hospitals. These wards were always recognised as places from which very few older people were ever discharged.

The people living in the local community often perceived the long-stay hospitals as being the end of the road for their relatives. The geriatric long-stay wards were poorly decorated and occupied by up to forty or more long-term patients who had reached their twilight years. Many of these patients suffered from a variety of conditions, including dementia. Patients were kept in their pyjamas all day with little or no stimulation, and were cared for by staff who suffered themselves from low wages, long hours and poor working conditions. In many cases, low staff morale was endemic throughout the wards.

Ward sisters and charge nurses were often limited in the supply of resources such as new furniture, coffee tables and televisions. Often it was left to the work of the hospital's League of Friends to raise charitable money to pay for perceived luxuries such as new televisions and video players for the patients' use. The League of Friends was made up of a dedicated group of well-meaning, hard-working local people who raised funds through organising bring and buy sales, car boot sales and summer fairs.

The long-stay ward day rooms had a small number of poorly-upholstered chairs which were placed around the walls. Patients had access to an old radio or a small television, which was switched on throughout the day and early evening until the patients were put to bed. The volume was usually very high and the music or programmes were often bland and repetitive. The television viewing was not the patients' choice, but often that of the staff on duty.

Patients' meals were often unappetising and presented in a way that didn't encourage anyone to look forward to meal times. The meals were often prepared in large hospital kitchens and then placed into large containers. These containers were towed around the hospital grounds by the hospital porters in large convoys of trucks. This transport system was fine in the summer months, but totally impractical in the winter when the food often reached the outlying wards only lukewarm, rather than piping hot. The nutritional value of meals was questionable, and cooked breakfasts disappeared from the menu in a cost-cutting exercise.

The general health of older people in hospital was poorly monitored due to lack of qualified staff. Inevitably, the scenes of desperation and, in some cases, lack of confidence were often witnessed throughout the National Health Service (NHS). I am convinced that this situation preyed on the minds of those people in power, whose responsibility it was to develop a new, efficient and more effective NHS.

Those with influence in government and public service unions suddenly began to realise that the general public would no longer tolerate the poor treatment of older people. Media coverage, including some high profile whistle blowing cases, resulted in a dramatic revolution which began to take place during the early 1970s.

The introduction of dedicated occupational therapists, medical consultants, physiotherapists and senior nurses demonstrated a personal commitment from professionals who had chosen to work and specialise in gerontology.

Suddenly many large independent care providers, builders and businessmen and women were encouraged to design and develop purpose built specialist care homes. These were to be situated in the local community and would cater for individuals with long-stay care needs.

This initiative allowed many local small NHS hospitals to close their long-stay wards. The majority of NHS staff had the opportunity to work in the independent sector for the first time. Individuals living in the new-style nursing homes were encouraged to wear their own clothes rather than nightclothes. The wearing of nightclothes during the day had sadly been regarded as normal and acceptable for many years in the long-stay wards. Older people were now to be provided with their own bedrooms. In some cases people were offered a shared twin bedroom, but by the end of the 1980s the emphasis was clearly moving towards providing people with their own single en-suite bedroom.

This change of emphasis and environment allowed many older people to move into the community and out of long-stay hospitals and marked the beginning of care homes as we know them today.

CHAPTER 1

SO YOU WANT TO BE A CARE HOME MANAGER?

Are you a self-motivated and experienced leader with a background working in care and do you wish to make a real difference to a group of older people's lives?

If you can answer 'yes' to these simple questions, then this book is for you.

Care home managers come from a variety of backgrounds and there comes a time in your career when you may decide to step up and apply to become a care home manager. Once you have made the decision, it is important to find the right care home manager's vacancy.

Ideally, you will possess management leadership qualities, including care experience, self-confidence and ambition. In *Nursing and Residential Care* (2003) Dr N. Chambers suggests that:

> *"The personal qualities which care home managers bring to the job are important, as well as the technical skills and expertise that they may possess."*

Care home managers must be capable of addressing the need to change. They must be willing to communicate the action plan formulated to manage the change to all the staff team. This will ensure that changes are made as part of a continuous and complex process.

WRITING YOUR CURRICULUM VITAE

Perhaps one of the most important records of your career to date is your personal curriculum vitae (CV). *In The Job Hunter's Handbook* (1999)

Greenwood reflects that:

> *"Curriculum Vitae is a Latin term which means 'the course of your life'. A good CV will be simple, short (two pages are usually sufficient, you can always compress or highlight details as necessary) and clear but it will be enough to enable an employer to see that you have the skills and qualities to match the job advertised".*

Whether you are considering moving to a new company or seeking internal promotion, it is advisable to prepare a well-presented up-to-date CV. Sometimes prospective employers may request a CV and covering letter before any short-listing takes place. On other occasions employers choose not to accept CVs but ask prospective candidates to complete a standard company application form. If you send out a CV that is not up-to-date, you send out a signal to the prospective employer that you are not really serious about wanting the post for which you have applied.

There are two important points that you should consider before you put together your CV.

- Do you have access to a complete and accurate record of your education and qualifications?
- Do you have access to a computer or know of someone who can type your CV?

The CV is the first opportunity you have to be short-listed for the job for which you have applied. Your CV should ensure that you stand out from the rest of the candidates.

In Nursing and Residential Care, October 2001, Sewell provides the following good advice:

> *"A CV should be written on clean, good quality paper, and it is better to choose a font that is clear and easy to read rather than something fancy and barely legible. Needless to say the CV should be grammatically correct and checked thoroughly for spelling mistakes".*

Personal details should include your address and contact details. People now give their personal email address, but it is inadvisable to give your present work number on your CV. Your educational details should be set out clearly. Include dates of courses undertaken and dates of any examination results. You may be asked at a later date for proof of examination results, so please do not make the grades higher than you achieved and remember that providing false information on a CV may result in a job offer being withdrawn.

Employment details should start with your present position. It is useful to put on record your responsibilities and achievements in each post.

Remember, while you have to sell yourself as well as you can, it is not a good idea to over-state your skills and attributes. When you are applying for a care home manager's post, there will be many other people in competition for it. An excellent CV will leave the prospective employer wanting to learn more about you.

Employers do want to know if you have any hobbies and interests, but if you list these, be ready for probing questions from the interview panel.

THE INTERVIEW PROCESS – A WINNING FORMULA

Attending interviews can be very stressful, not only for the candidates but also for those people involved in the interview process. As a candidate you must be prepared for a variety of questions and scenarios, not only on clinical issues but also on business related matters concerning the care home.

Your appearance is a vital part of your preparation, as first impressions are so important. Consider the interview process has started when you arrive and first speak to the receptionist at the centre where the interview is taking place. In some cases the managing director of the care company may seek the personal observations of the reception staff about each of the candidates.

It is essential to research the care home manager's role and you should find out some information about the care home. You may find information on the company's web site by using the internet. If you do your research, you will have a good idea of the sort of questions that the panel may ask.

Be clear and concise with your answers and do not waffle. If you are not sure of an answer, then tell the panel. Honesty is always the best policy.

Remember not to undersell yourself, but be aware of the danger of over- promoting your skills. Employers are looking for people with whom they can work in the future. It may be that you have all the right qualifications but the wrong sort of personality for the specific role they have in mind.

Eye contact and body language are important, as the panel members will be watching candidates' behaviour. Some companies invite the candidates for lunch and this is commonly known as "trial by sherry". In other cases, people may be asked for interviews over two days and this method of selection will include psychometric testing, group work, presentations and role-play. If you are asked to give your personal views on topical care issues of the day, then ensure that you answer honestly.

From the first moment of contact with the potential employer and as the interview moves forward, each panel member is forming an opinion as to your suitability for the position of care home manager. Today many short-listed candidates are asked to give a short presentation at interview on a given subject. Therefore it is really useful to have an understanding and working knowledge of PowerPoint.

Preparing PowerPoint Presentations

Care home managers may be called upon to give presentations at their interview. This is important because, once appointed, the successful candidate may be asked to present in-house training sessions for staff.

PowerPoint is a computer software programme which allows you to make professional slide presentations and display the results on a portable screen via a special projector. Alternatively, you can display the slide show using a normal laptop computer if there is only a small number of people to view the presentation. Sound can be added to the transition between slides.

Step-by-step guidelines to successful presentation

1. Choose the template. This will be seen on all slides.
2. Choose the individual slide layout.
3. Choose clip art or pictures. These images will enhance your presentation.
4. Choose the text. Keep this simple, no more than seven words per sentence.
5. Text can be displayed line by line or all at once.
6. Choose transition between slides and then practise slide show.

7. The slide show can be as short or as long as you like, but the average number of slides in a presentation is between 16 and 20.

Remember that people no longer expect to see presentations done with the use of overhead projectors and acetates; they have come to accept PowerPoint as the new standard to which we all must aspire. The computer will guide you through the formulation of your slide show, but I urge you to try this simple system for yourself. In my personal opinion, PowerPoint presentations are now seen as the normal method of visual communication.

CHAPTER 2

THE CARE HOME MANAGER'S ROLE

In Nursing and Residential Care (2003) Chambers acknowledges that:

> *"Well run care homes depend crucially on the skills and leadership attributes of the managers. Their role often combines that of lead clinician, operational manager, finance manager, marketing director and advocate for residents and staff."*

Today the care home manager has a demanding and satisfying role both from a care and business perceptive. The principal responsibility is to ensure that individuals always receive excellent standards of high quality care and service while they are accommodated in the care home of their choice. This high quality care can only be delivered if the home is well staffed with appropriately trained and highly motivated personnel. Care home managers appear as the conductors of their orchestras, and their ability to keep all the facilities and staff members operating successfully takes special skills and knowledge. This makes such posts the most demanding in care today.

EXAMPLE OF A CARE HOME MANAGER'S JOB DESCRIPTION

Position: care home manager

Responsible to: regional manager

- Responsibility for the day-to-day management of the care home.
- To achieve and maintain high standards of care.
- To meet regulatory obligations.
- To meet and try and exceed budgetary targets.
- To train and develop staff team members.

- Philosophy
- To provide individual older people with quality long-term care.
- To meet and exceed the individuals' needs in a cost-effective manner.
- To involve relatives and friends with individuals' activities both inside the care home and in the local community.
- To be a personal ambassador and role model for staff team members.

- Standards of care
- Ensure that the operational policies and procedures are carried out in accordance with the company's expected high standard.
- Ensure that all staff team members are fully trained in the correct methods of delivering of care for older people.

- Produce staff rotas ensuring adequate staffing levels with the right skill mix.
- Personally monitor clinical and business standards throughout the care home.
- Notify the regional manager within 24 hours of any untoward incident or complaint, irrespective of its source.
- Notify the regional manager of any serious accident or contagious illness; confirm the actions you have taken by fax or e-mail.
- Ensure that each resident has an individualised care plan. Monitor care plans to make sure they are being implemented properly.
- Identify therapeutic activity programmes.

■ Regulatory and statutory obligations

- Ensure compliance with regulatory and statutory obligations.
- Maintain satisfactory relationships with the CSCI inspectorate, purchasers of care and other outside agencies.
- Be acutely aware of any proposed legislation changes which may affect the business and the manager's role.

■ Profitability

- Maximise revenue by optimising the number of individuals' fees wherever possible.
- Minimise debts through timely action.
- Ensure staff hours and costs are within agreed limits.
- Control expenditure to ensure best price and purchase orders are authorised
- Ensure control and reconciliation of petty cash and individual residents' personal monies.

- Work with regional manager to develop annual budget in line with company's expectations.

- Staffing issues
- Be involved in the recruitment and selection of all staff within the care home in conjunction with human resources department.
- Ensure that members of the staff team are competent, trained and perform to the best of their abilities.
- Carry out disciplinary action in accordance with the company's procedure.
- Adhere to the company's employment policies.
- Advise the regional manager of potential staff problems.

- Administration and other duties
- Ensure that all administrative and accounting tools are effectively used.
- Ensure that all returns are forwarded to head office accurately and on time.
- Ensure that building maintenance programmes are carried out satisfactorily.
- Ensure all medication is adequately controlled and the required records are kept.
- Ensure that the care home is promoted within the local community.
- Implement the agreed marketing plan.
- Carry out any other duties as discussed with the regional manager.

PERSONAL PROFILE FOR MANAGERS IN THE FUTURE

The perfect profile for a care home manager is well-documented, but I have devised my own profile based on personal experience.

Professional qualification

The care home manager may have undertaken nursing studies and achieved a recognised nursing qualification. The manager will have also undertaken the registered manager's award NVQ level 4 and will ideally be a qualified NVQ assessor. Before anyone is appointed as a care home manager they should have at least two years' experience in managing within the independent care sector.

Professional qualifications are important, but the strength and qualities of managers can be developed once they have been appointed to take charge of a home. This requires the support and guidance of a regional operations manager within larger companies, or the sole proprietor of a smaller company. Working in the NHS cannot adequately prepare staff for becoming successful care home managers, and it is only once in post that managers realise the true reality and scope of the position.

Gone are the days when sole proprietors of care homes took charge of everything apart from the bedside care. Care home managers need to be multi-skilled and to have the ability to lead a team of people who can together achieve a successful and profitable business operation. The following are attributes needed by those aspiring to become effective care home managers of the future.

Honesty

Care home managers have a personal responsibility for dealing with the residents' finances and are trusted to act in the resident's best interest at all times (Department of Health 2000). Handling large amounts of other people's money carries with it a burden of responsibility, and the internal systems adopted by the care home manager must be seen to be transparent and stand the scrutiny of any unannounced internal or external audit process.

There needs to be a recognised method of recording any transactions involving money and it is essential that receipts are kept.

Name of resident	Gladys Smith Date of Birth: 25th February 1930			
Date	**Money taken out**	**Money remaining in account**	**Signature resident**	**Signature carer**
12th March	£20.00	£40.00		
18th March	£10.00	£30.00		
21st March	£5.00	£25.00		
24th March	£10.00	£15.00		
All receipts must be kept in the resident's account box which must be kept in the safe				

As care home managers are communicating every day with staff and outside agencies at all levels, their honesty and integrity must be beyond reproach. Relatives and residents have the right to receive information which is honest, factual and delivered without prejudice.

Well-organised

Care home managers need to be organised in order that they can control the clinical and financial performance of their home. A well-organised care home manager will often introduce and maintain a strict discipline and routine for the rest of the staff to follow. Clear objectives will be produced for the team so that they can achieve outstanding results.

In Organise Yourself (2000) Caunt recommends that you should

> *"Try to produce objectives that are SMART – Specific, Measurable, Achievable, Result-orientated and Time-related".*

The care home manager's personal management style can be witnessed from the moment any visitor enters the reception area of the care home. A well-organised care home manager will always ensure that all residents' files, staff personnel documentation, miscellaneous records and service contracts are filed in locked cabinets. If there is an efficient filing system in place with easy access for authorised staff, the well-organised manager can find any document requested in minutes.

Caunt (2000) also reflects that:

> *"Much of our working day is spent in some form of interaction with others. The way you approach these interactions can have a considerable impact on your effectiveness".*

On the other hand, the disorganised care home manager can never seem to find any document and appears to work in a cluttered and untidy office with no visible filing system in place.

Often the appointment of a good care home administrator can be the first step in assisting the care home manager to achieve a more efficient approach to the role. The role of the administrator should never be underestimated, but it is the home manager who ultimately has the responsibility for ensuring the care home is managed as well as possible.

Clinically skilled

Nurses and carers with high levels of clinical skill are often reluctant to move into management, but sometimes clinicians can become excellent leaders and care home managers within the independent care sector. Clinical skills are important if the care home manager is to establish a model of care within the establishment and hopes to change the way things are done.

Staff team members will have more respect for a care home manager with a relevant background, clinical knowledge and hands-on experience in a specialist field of care, rather than for someone with a general caring background and no specific specialist skills. It is essential that the care home manager has experience in writing and implementing individualised care plans which demonstrate his or her clinical expertise.

Experience in the field

Care home managers need to have experience in the field they choose to operate in, and the more practical experience they have the better. It is difficult to imagine a care home manager with little or no experience in dementia care running a well-established centre for older people with dementia. If care home managers can demonstrate to staff their levels of experience, then it will be easier to motivate staff to encompass the change of practices that may be necessary to move the care home forward.

Excellent communication

The care home manager needs to possess excellent communication skills, both verbal and written. Managers need to be computer-literate and should be able to use e-mails and the internet.

Much of the care home manager's day-to-day routine is spent

talking to people, including potential residents and their families. The care home manager should have a professional but friendly disposition and be able to put people at their ease. A warm and caring welcome is of paramount importance when meeting people who visit the home, or in meetings elsewhere. The way people are approached can affect the way they respond, and the care home manager should set a good example to all staff as to how people should be addressed. A care home manager must treat people with respect in order to gain respect.

A sense of humour

Individuals working in care spend many hours in stressful situations. The care home manager who has a good sense of humour can often defuse potential confrontational issues in the care home. Having a sense of humour does not just mean always seeing the funny side of issues but, more importantly, maintaining empathy with the rest of the team and striking a balance between being seen as a well-rounded individual or a standoffish person. There are many funny things that happen in care homes, and things that residents say often bring a welcome smile to people's faces.

Highly-motivated

A highly-motivated and enthusiastic care home manager often encourages other staff members to raise the level of their performance. The ability to motivate others is a wonderful skill and should always be sought as a necessary attribute when appointing any new care home manager. In *How to Motivate People* (2000) Forsyth suggests that:

> *"Almost every activity a manager engages in will have motivational consequences... What makes people good and positive about their employer, particularly their manager, and above all their job and all it entails. And what creates negative feelings?...Motivation*

demands honesty and sincerity. It is very difficult to motivate if in truth, you do not really care about people."

Motivational skills can be taught, but the secret of success is for the care home manager to really care about each member of staff. Once the staff recognise this, they will follow the manager no matter how tough the journey.

Showing initiative

Successful care home managers are those who are able to assess a situation and provide a solution to any problem. They must have the ability to develop a robust action plan and implement the actions of the staff team in order to achieve the required outcome. This outcome needs to be within budget and in line with the companies overall objectives.

Self-motivation is having the confidence to be pro-active, rather than being re-active and waiting for others to initiate change. Self-starters are usually first on duty and last off, because they know how important it is to set the right example to others.

Have vision and values

Strong leaders will inspire those around them to achieve their maximum potential and strive for excellence. In *Making it Happen – Reflections on Leadership* (1989) Harvey-Jones reflects:

"One of the lessons I have learnt in life is that a little bit more time thinking and planning, will immeasurably increase the effectiveness of one's input".

Delivering outstanding service and care needs to be managed at all levels. While all staff may not possess the same levels of skills and commitment, it remains the care home manager's responsibility to ensure that the company's vision and values are carried through in all aspects of running the care home. People who are employed in the care home must buy into the culture of the company and believe in the way the care home is being developed.

Strong leaders empower those who work with them to deliver the results. Care home managers are only as good as the teams they build around them.

Physically fit

Care home managers need to be physically fit, as the hours they work would otherwise have an adverse effect on their health. It is important that any medical concerns they have disclosed at interview should be addressed quickly. Sometimes, after managers are appointed, they find that they cannot cope with the demands of the job due to an underlying health condition. Health screening is very important and many companies now provide care home managers with private health care insurance cover as part of their employment package.

Managers who are overweight may face potential health problems. The image portrayed is very important, especially in prestigious care homes where people are often judged by the way they look and not by how good they are at doing the job. While this common prejudice cannot be condoned, it is sadly a fact of modern life. In some areas there are cases of ageism. This should always be discouraged, as many mature people are physically and mentally fit for the role of care home manager.

A good role model

Care home managers must be aware of their personal behaviour both in work and outside work. This may appear very harsh, but the managers have the reputations of their care homes to consider, and while they are out in the community they are acting as ambassadors for their homes. People are very quick to criticise, and managers should be aware of their professional responsibilities.

Excellent attendance record

Managers with poor attendance records may find it difficult to discipline staff team members if they themselves are always off sick with a variety of ailments. People accept those with genuine ill health, but some staff do appear to take advantage and seem to be under the false impression that they have a right to a certain amount of sick leave on an annual basis.

Customer-focused

Care home managers who are customer-focussed are able to demonstrate this clearly by adopting the three As principles of customer care. These are Attitude, Appearance and Approach. Successful care home managers always have positive attitudes and they are clear about meeting and exceeding the customer's expectations. They know their internal and external customers' needs.

Care home managers who have a pride in their appearance reflect a positive image for the rest of the home. Staff throughout the home will also take pride in their personal appearance because the manager always looks smart and wears the uniform correctly.

The care home manager should always present a professional approach to everyone within the care home. Individual residents, visitors and staff must be treated consistently with good manners and a caring nature.

An innovator

Care home managers who are innovators are usually very keen to introduce new ideas, but only after they have researched them and discussed them with the rest of the team. It is often disastrous to try and introduce change unilaterally, and many newly-appointed managers have fallen by the wayside because they have tried to introduce changes without the support of their staff. Consultation and discussions with staff at all levels are vital if new ideas are to be implemented successfully.

Business awareness

Care home managers must have a clear and up-to-date knowledge of budgets and the terminology used when discussing profit and loss, accounts, and balance sheets. Care home managers must be aware of the need to make a profit in order to invest money back into the care home and to be able to meet the wages and overheads of running the business.

It is easy to try and leave this responsibility to someone else, but ultimately the buck stops with the manager and the care home's success or failure lies with them. Likewise, it is important to address the marketing of the home and be aware of the competition in the local area or nationally, depending upon which type of services is being provided.

Strategic thinker

The care home manager is responsible for implementing the company's strategic business plan. While it is recognised that the company's strategic business plan is based on short-, medium- and long-term objectives, in reality most care home managers are concerned with dealing with the short-term consequences of their home's occupancy, fee levels and resource management.

Achieving a work - life balance

Today many care home managers are expected to be on call 24 hours a day and may be contacted at home in an emergency. Care home managers who are always available can make rods for their own backs. However, some care home managers want to know everything and would be displeased if they were not contacted when an incident happened in the home. It is important that care home managers strike a balance between their personal and working lives.

THE SMALL BUSINESS GROWTH

In *Exploring Corporate Strategy* (1993) Johnson and Scholes state:

> *"For a small business a major issue is the management of growth. Successful small businesses grow out of the founder's entrepreneurial vision, but growth means the founder can no longer manage all the activities alone."*

Care home managers who work for a small group of care homes may find themselves facing major change and restructure as the small group begins to grow. It is extremely important to ensure that all staff are involved in the change of culture from the corner shop to the supermarket as this is a complex process.

RESPONSIBILITIES OF THE CARE HOME MANAGER

- To maximise bed occupancy and establish the care home's fee structure in line with the company's expectations.
- To agree, develop and implement the care home's annual budget.

- To control the care home's direct costs in line with the agreed annual budget.
- To control the care home's operating costs, including wage costs.
- To ensure that the overheads are monitored and efficiently used in line with agreed budgeted forecasts.
- To ensure that the recruitment and selection of staff team members is carried out in line with the company's agreed protocol and procedures.
- To undertake in-house training for all grades of staff and partake in supervision and appraisals as and when agreed with the company.
- To ensure that clinical and social activities are based on best practice.
- To ensure that all staff adhere to the home's policies and procedures.
- To ensure that the care home is fit for purpose and meets the standards set out in the Care Standards Act 2000 and inspection process carried out by CSCI.
- To follow up any CSCI recommendations and requirements within the agreed time frame.
- To report and document any accidents or untoward incidents in the agreed manner.
- To liaise with relatives and staff by holding regular information meetings and to keep a detailed record of the minutes of these meetings followed up with a robust action plan.

ADMINISTRATION, ORDERING AND STORAGE OF MEDICINES

The care home manager must ensure that all qualified staff undertake personal and professional training in order to protect individual residents and colleagues with regard to the procurement, storage, administration, recording and disposal of all medicines. These procedures must be carried out in a professional manner, complying with the agreed National Minimum Care Standards and the care home's policies and procedures. While undertaking an internal audit of the care home, the local pharmacist will expect any issues raised in previous visits to have been addressed and rectified by the care home manager. It is good practice to communicate in writing the actions taken, not only to the local pharmacist but also to the CSCI homes' inspectorate.

Local care homes' policies and procedures must be adhered to at all times. From time to time it may be necessary for the care home's policies and procedures to be reviewed and updated. This is the personal responsibility of the care home manager in consultation with the local pharmacist. Any changes must be communicated to all staff, both verbally and in writing, to avoid any confusion arising at a later stage. The following issues may be covered during the internal audit.

Security of Medicines

The drugs room in which the medicines are stored must be kept locked when not in use and the windows must be secured. The storage cupboards must be fixed to a load-bearing wall, not a partition wall. These must be locked and the person in charge of each shift must hold the keys to this room. The medicine trolley must be locked and fixed to a load-bearing wall when not in use.

Hazard notices

A dated record must be kept of actions taken against all hazard notices received by the care home. It is important to record what action you have taken against each of the hazard notices issued.

Prescribing and recording medicines

- The care home manager must ensure that the general practitioner (GP) writes individual residents' prescriptions using a Form FP10.
- A photocopy of the FP10 should be kept in the resident's file for a minimum of three months. A method of recording all the medicines received from the local pharmacy by the care home must be in place.
- Medicines are supplied to the care home from the nominated pharmacy in response to the individual resident's FP10.
- All medicines issued are supplied for an individually-named resident. The blister pack will be labelled with the resident's name, full directions for use and the date dispensed.
- All medicines received in the care home must be checked by a qualified nurse or a senior carer in a residential setting. This staff member is responsible for checking each medication against the photocopied FP10 and enters it on the individual's audit sheet and Medication Administration Record (MAR) sheet.
- Medicines must be stored in the appropriate drug cupboard, trolley or special lockable drugs refrigerator.
- The care home manager must make weekly checks of the drug cupboard, or a designated first level qualified nurse, or senior carer in a residential setting must record their findings in the weekly checks book, located in the drugs room.
- When a resident is admitted from home, hospital or any other place, the nurse in charge, or the senior carer in a residential setting, ascertains that the medicines appear fit for use and appropriately labelled. The resident's GP is informed and new medicines are prescribed using an FP10.
- A record must be kept on the audit sheet or MAR sheet of all medicines which, when no longer in use, are returned

to the pharmacy for safe disposal. A signature from the pharmacist acknowledging safe receipt is required.

Controlled drugs

- The controlled drugs book or CD book must be kept up to date and include a list of signatures of staff who are responsible for the administration of medicines in the home.
- The controlled drugs must be stored in a locked cupboard within a locked cupboard.
- All controlled drugs disposed of must be collected by the pharmacist and recorded in the retail pharmacist's register or disposal record book.
- It is the responsibility of care home managers to spot-check controlled drug books and the stock levels at any time and record their findings.

Administration of medicines

- The monitored dosage system implemented in many care homes throughout the United Kingdom use forms known as Medication Administration Record (MAR sheets).
- The MAR sheet is generated following the receipt by the pharmacist of an FP10 prescription written and authorised by the GP. The pharmacist dispenses and delivers the medicines to the care home and these are checked upon arrival by a qualified nurse or, in a residential setting, by the person in charge of the shift. A record is made to state that the medicines have been accepted into the care home.
- The MAR sheets are used to record the medications administered for individual residents.
- An up-to-date photograph of each client must accompany the MAR sheet. Identification of individuals is of

paramount importance, and is especially useful for agency staff, who may only spend one shift in the care home.

- Check that the name on the bottle or blister pack corresponds to the name on the MAR sheet.
- A first or second level nurse, or a senior carer in a residential setting, administers the medicines at the prescribed times to the individual residents and signs either the drug chart or the MAR sheet, once they are sure that the individual resident has taken the medication.
- If for any reason the medicine is not given, then the appropriate code should be entered in place of the nurse's signature located on the MAR sheet or drug chart.
- Controlled drugs are administered and entered into the controlled drugs book and there must always be a witness signature, which does not have to be a first level nurse.
- Homely remedies are medications approved by the GP for occasional use by the residents, but not ordered using an FP10.
- A list of homely remedies should be displayed in the drugs room. Remedies are recorded as having been administered on the drugs chart or MAR sheet and the homely remedies book.
- Homely remedies should be purchased by the home and stored in the drug trolley and marked 'Homely Remedies'.
- The administration of medicines may be observed from time to time by the care home manager to ensure that medicines are being administered correctly in line with local policies and procedures.
- It is important that stock levels are checked regularly as sometimes staff do over-order and stockpile. This is especially the case with lotions.
- Care home managers should adopt a 'just in time' policy which ensures that stock levels are always adequate but never excessive.
- Care home managers using the MDS system order the residents' medications on a specific day for the next 28

days. All stock must be accounted for and if a medicine is no longer required, then this should be made clear, to both the GP and the pharmacist.

- Surplus stock on the shelves equates to money spent and has a direct impact on achieving a balanced budget. This affects the GP's budget but not the care home's.
- Care home managers must ensure that any residents wishing to self-medicate have their medicines dispensed by the retail pharmacist and stored in a locked cupboard within their own room.
- Following a risk assessment carried out by the named nurse, the resident may be given access to a key to their medicine storage box within their own room. However, weekly checks should be carried out by the qualified nurse to ensure the resident's compliance with the prescription.
- The care home manager should undertake an audit of the medicines and the MAR sheets at least once a month.

Storage of medicines

Managers should ensure internal and external medicines are stored separately and labelled correctly. Storage of medicines is very important, as there may be medicines which need to be stored in a refrigerator. The drugs fridge should be checked regularly to ensure the thermostat is working correctly. The refrigerator should be defrosted regularly and kept locked when not in use. Staff should be encouraged to keep the refrigerator clean and tidy. It is important that the room allocated to storing the medicines is always locked when not in use. The person in charge of the shift should hold the medicine keys. Staff must not store any other equipment in the room designated for the storage of medicines.

Storage and use of medical gases

Within the care home there must be a safe place to store oxygen cylinders. It is important that empty oxygen cylinders are replaced as quickly as is practicable. They need to be kept securely to avoid accidents and a sign must be displayed warning clients' relatives and any other visitors about the strict No Smoking policy in or around storage areas.

All staff should be trained in the administration of oxygen and residents must always have the oxygen prescribed by the GP before administration.

Pharmaceutical advice

A successful care home manager will build a good working relationship with the local pharmacist in order to ensure that prescriptions are despatched on time. It is also important that there is a good communication network built up between the GP, staff members and the local pharmacist.

The pharmacist is available to give advice and may be able to offer staff training. He or she may be able to work alongside the manager in order to audit the performance of the home with regard to maintaining a high standard of medicine administration. A safe and secure systematic approach to this function is fundamental to the smooth running of any care home.

Members of staff's approach and delivery of the medicines is often indicative of the level of overall service delivery that may be expected throughout the rest of the home. The medicine records must be accurate and up-to-date, and the number of errors needs to be examined closely to avoid recurrence. A consistent approach to the administration of medicines can, in my view, help reduce the risk of drug errors occurring.

Evidence of on-going staff development and training and monitoring of drug procedures by the care home manager will help demonstrate the commitment to maintaining high standards, ensuring that clients are given their medication appropriately and correctly. Staff must be encouraged to demonstrate discipline and pay great attention to detail.

Care home managers must appreciate that they have a personal duty of care to individual residents and ensure that all staff are appropriately trained, supervised and monitored in the correct administration of medicines.

Managing staff from overseas

There has been a dramatic increase in the number of qualified staff from overseas, and they have brought a new and fresh perspective to the care business. The overseas staff bring with them their individual cultures, music and spiritual values which can be a valuable asset to many care homes.

A care home manager should endeavour to make the transition into the local community and integration into the care team as smooth as possible.

Responsibility for staff training

Care home managers today are faced with many diverse issues. These may include the necessity to fill the beds and keep overheads to a minimum in line with the agreed budget, whilst meeting the requirements of the national minimum care standards. These can be found by visiting www.dh.gov.uk.

The criterion for any successful manager is to fill beds, deliver excellent care utilising resources efficiently and effectively, and thus encouraging people to want to buy the services on offer. This develops the need for a waiting list; the good care homes get better and the poor homes start to slide into extinction.

Investment in the training of all staff is of paramount importance. The manager needs to be able to teach, but should also be authorised to buy in training from specialist companies. These will deliver statutory and NVQ training which remain at the centre of the present government's strategy to improve care standards throughout the country.

Empowering staff

The staff are the greatest asset in any care home, and if they are allowed to develop to meet and exceed their personal aspirations, then the home will become successful with an enhanced reputation in the community.

In *The Power of Empowerment* (1994) Clutterbuck offers several definitions of empowerment:

- *"Encouraging and allowing individuals to take personal responsibility for improving the way they do their jobs and contribute to the company's goals. It requires the creation of a culture which both encourages people at all levels to feel that they can make a difference, and helps them to acquire the confidence and skills to do so."*

Clutterbuck further explains that the concept of empowerment is often resisted for the following reasons:

- *"People are wary of change.*
- *Many employees have reason to be sceptical of empowerment.*
- *Not everyone wants to be empowered."*

Managers are therefore responsible for making sure they recognise potential in all staff members, irrespective of their position within the care home. It is simple to see the senior staff becoming empowered, but empowerment is also important for junior members of staff. For empowerment to take place, managers should recognise members of staff's individual strengths and their aptitude for the role envisaged for them in the home. It is not enough to guess what people are capable of, so this process will entail a certain amount of consultation.

Managers must be able to delegate key tasks, and giving staff certain levels of responsibility gives them a sense of well-being and encourages them to give more of themselves to enhance the development of the team, thereby improving the quality of care clients receive. Staff who are empowered appear much more motivated than staff who are kept in check by managers displaying an autocratic management style. People respond positively to being allowed to take initiative.

An improved quality of life for residents is of paramount importance, whether they are elderly or young people with a physical disability. There are a number of simple ways in which both clients and staff can be empowered in the care centre.

The staff and residents' forum

In some care homes there are residents' and relatives' committees which provide a platform for residents and their families to discuss the care and activities available in the home. These meetings are designed to allow people to air their personal viewpoints without fear of repercussion. The chairperson should be the care home manager, who will in turn investigate any issues that are raised and attempt to provide solutions.

In order to create active partnerships in care, there must always be the opportunity for honest and open channels of communication.

A meeting of staff chaired by the home manager or a senior member of staff helps to plan and implement an agenda for change. Organising outings for staff and clients may involve a great deal of additional effort, but the rewards can be effectively measured in the clients' individual responses to their improved activities. Older people need to be encouraged to partake in physical, social and stimulating activities.

The response of staff to organised activities can be an encouragement to clients. If staff show no interest in organised activities and outings, then getting the clients to be enthusiastic is almost impossible. A highly motivated manager leading staff from the front will have a positive effect on the morale of staff and clients alike. It is important to have support from relatives as their involvement may encourage the quieter clients to take part. In the past, due to their personalities, these residents may not have taken part in any activities.

Recently a large care company purchased people carriers for a number of their care homes. The response from staff and residents was excellent and the clients enjoyed being able to make summer visits to different locations.

Day-care facilities attached to a care home can offer opportunities to older people who live alone in their own homes in the community. They will be able to undertake activities in a warm and secure environment with people of their own age and similar interests.

Social isolation and loneliness means that many older people do not have the chance to talk to anyone, sometimes for days on end. However, the introduction of day-care allows that cycle of depression to be broken, and thankfully managers can ensure that their clients need not suffer the same fate.

The care home manager can ensure that clients are escorted into the local community either in the home's transport or on foot, if the weather is favourable and depending on the proximity of the home to the local amenities. Shopping trips and theatre and cinema visits should be seen as normal for clients and not as the exception to the rule. Informed choice for individuals means that they will be able to choose what activities they would like to undertake to improve their quality of life.

Clients' relationships

Inevitably, some clients who are living in a care centre may have an opportunity to begin a new relationship and, while their families should be informed about any relationships, staff should be non-judgemental and should facilitate the elderly to ensure they live as normally as possible. This sensitive area is a real part of long-term care which is often avoided.

Managers must be aware of the possibilities that clients may fall in love, and how they deal with these situations can have a dramatic impact in the smooth running of the home.

In *Sexuality and Residential Care: Issues for Staff and Clients* (2001) Penhale and Manthorpe state that

> *"Staff can get caught up in issues such as 'whether older people have sexual needs' or 'how to best allow individuals to fulfil their sexual needs, and with whom'. There may be further areas of concern such as how to be sure that there is mutual consent within a relationship which has developed where some residents are particularly frail, and whose rights (if anyone's) should take precedence within situations that develop".*

Informed choice for both clients and staff allows people to take decisions which improve their individual lives.

Communication

Open and honest communication is very important between all parties, including staff, family and the social worker, in assisting clients to improve their lives. Arranging supported holidays for clients is seen not as a luxury, but as an integral part of their lives. Through the last two decades many people who are reaching pensionable age will have spent most of their adult lives enjoying foreign holidays.

The care home manager has a responsibility to ensure that the client's holiday plans are discussed with family members and to agree the location, cost of holiday and type of holiday. A list of holidays should be kept in the care home.

CHAPTER 3

REFLECTIVE PRACTICE

All managers and staff have a personal responsibility to reflect on all aspects of their professional practice. Qualified nurses in particular are encouraged to reflect on their practice as part of their personal development.

Reflective practice consists of cognitive activities, such as comparing and contrasting phenomena, recognising patterns, categorising perceptions, framing and self-questioning, in order to create meaning and understanding.

Self-questioning is a significant process within reflective thinking. Three hierarchical levels of reflective thinking have been identified:

- Reflective thinking-for-action centres on the current situation.
- Reflective thinking-for-evaluation focuses on creating wholeness and contributes to the realisation of multiple perceptions and multiple responses.
- Reflective thinking-for-critical inquiry, which is not widely used in nursing.

It is important for people to reflect on their practice for the following reasons:

- To evaluate the causes, effects and outcomes of their interactions with clients, relatives and staff on a regular basis.
- To keep an accurate record of good practice.

- To share experiences with other staff and broaden personal knowledge concerning developments in clinical and managerial practice.

Care workers and qualified nursing staff may be required to keep written evidence of how they transfer their underpinning knowledge of care into practice, either while undertaking an NVQ or NMC post-registration education and practice requirements (PREP).

The elements of reflective practice are easy to follow:

Personal notes

Once the care home manager and staff begin to reflect on their individual practice, they will find that writing personal notes becomes an integral part of this important exercise.

Historically, nurses have often struggled with the thought of having to write their interventions down and in many cases they claim they have no time. There are many interruptions in their busy schedules. The care plans of residents are a legal document, but personal reflective diaries are meant to act as an aide-memoire for individual staff members.

Personal notes are a permanent record of what has happened, how an issue was addressed and what the outcome was. Once this is written down it can be re-visited and used as evidence if an issue recurs. Some staff choose to transfer their notes onto their personal computer or laptop. The way the information is stored should be easily accessible, but protected by a password to prevent others from reading the material.

All personal notes should be dated and should not be used as part of any other documentation. In order to ensure confidentiality, it is vital that staff do not use clients' real names. Therefore staff should use initials or a false name to protect vulnerable clients and their families.

In order to practise the technique of keeping personal records, it is useful to choose a significant event and consider ways in which the situation was addressed, the time taken to deal with the matter and the outcome of the issue.

It is interesting to consider alternative ways in which the matter might have been handled and how the outcome might have been changed.

Thoughts

Thinking seriously about the results of a personal action regarding clients and their relatives may lead to a positive change in the future. However, before taking any course of action it is important to think clearly about the worst possible consequence of anything we do or say. During verbal exchanges managers must remain professional and diplomatic and ensure that they give both parties the opportunity to state their case. The danger is that people who are complaining believe that the manager will always believe and support the staff member. Complaints are remembered by those affected for many years and can damage and affect a manager's confidence. In some extreme cases people's careers are affected.

Relatives' feelings may change, given time, understanding and an opportunity to consider other people's point of view. The documentation collected is vital and it is important that any statements made are examined by the investigating officer. In some cases another care home manager may act as the investigating officer.

Criticism and complaints about staff and managers are often taken personally, even when they may believe that they did their best for the client.

The importance of keeping factual reports about relatives' and clients' concerns and complaints cannot be stressed strongly enough. In addition to the home's complaints book, managers should be mindful of keeping statements from staff and these should be kept in the client's notes. Today people are very keen to seek financial compensation whenever they have a grievance, and if the staff do not have accurate records of incidents and events, then they have no evidence of taking the correct action. Remember to report the following elements of any incident:

- When did the incident occur? Time and date are critical in this aspect of the record.
- Where did the incident happen? The location may prove critical in establishing the effect the incident had, not only on the client but on other clients and staff.
- Why did the incident happen? Often there are behavioural issues concerning certain clients.
- How was the incident dealt with? Was the care home manager involved and when were the relatives informed?
- What action has been taken to prevent the incident happening again?
- What lessons have been learned and does the home need to review any policies and procedures in order to safeguard clients or staff in the future?

The following incident illustrates only too well how important proper record-keeping is. A woman complained that her husband was dressed in another resident's trousers. She was very upset and the care home manager apologised and promised to sort the matter out. It transpired that the care home laundry had suffered a break down, so clothing had been taken to the launderette for drying. There was a delay in repairing the faulty machine, and other relatives started to complain about the state of the residents' clothes. Care home staff didn't want to co-operate with the launderette solution. In retrospect, the regional manager thought he should have hired a large dryer for the home instead of using the launderette.

This anecdote illustrates how a seemingly simple incident can escalate, and if each stage isn't recorded, it is very difficult for people to remember accurately what happened.

Building relationships

Only a few days after an individual resident's admission to the care home, if things are not going well then family members may start to express their concerns about the level of care their relative is receiving. Frustration may build up between the family and the care staff, and unless the issues are tackled and solutions found there may be some animosity demonstrated to various members of care staff.

Sometimes there may have been a great deal of soul-searching prior to agreeing to place an older relative in a local care home, and the guilt felt by the close family may result in a the family demonstrating a sensitive and demanding approach. Some people complain in order to ensure that their relative receives a high standard of care. Families who complain can be very personal in their criticism and staff need to be able to deal with the emotional outbursts.

Tackling the difficult customer

In *Managing difficult people* (2000) Mannering explains that there are some simple techniques to bear in mind when facing a difficult complainant:

> *"Try to ascertain their name early in the conversation and continue to use it throughout, let them know your name and position, maintain eye contact at all times and use positive body language (sitting forward, interested expression).*
>
> *Do not be bullied into resolving the problem immediately if you are unsure: however, promise a speedy response and give a date for settlement of the issue."*

Personal Reflection

When care staff are reflecting after duty they need time to relax and unwind. A partner who understands can help in this process and it is important to share thoughts about what can be a very stressful situation. However, it is important to remember to keep confidential information to yourself. Therefore no individuals should be mentioned by name. Staff failing to discuss issues with those people closest to them may damage their personal relationships.

Communication is vital in the reflection process. Those care home managers who do not talk through their worries and anxieties often store up trouble for themselves in the future.

Giving feedback

Again, in *Managing difficult people* (2000) Mannering urges the reader to:

> *"Remember – Ninety nine per cent of all difficult feedback is not intended to force a resignation. It is simply to improve performance, and it is important that this message is conveyed."*

Everyone appreciates positive feedback and staff must be made to feel comfortable and at ease in the work place. Working in a care home can be stressful and being a care home manager can be extremely stressful. Staff must support each other rather than conspiring to work against each other, which does happen in some care homes.

The effective care home manager will always try and balance good and bad news, but will try to ensure that team members are given the opportunity to receive the good news last.

Life-long learning

Staff need to talk through their own personal thoughts and feelings about their work, discussing the stresses and strains they experience.

An experienced care home manager or senior care support worker acting as mentor can encourage such discussion. Used in conjunction with reflection, these one-to-one sessions can prove most beneficial to both the manager and the staff member. Learning is a lifelong experience and therefore it is extremely important that staff have the chance to talk things through with a senior person.

We never stop learning, and as the role of the care home manager develops over the forthcoming years, successful care home managers will adapt in the best way they can to face the future.

Care home managers often feel isolated if they are part of a large group. However, it is possible to find support by contacting the Registered Nursing Home Association at www.rnha.co.uk. The RNHA was formed in 1968 and it campaigns strongly for high standards in nursing home care. Members are nursing home care owners and are committed to delivering quality services. The

RNHA can be contacted by email at info@rnha.co.uk.

Counsel and Care is a charity giving advice and information to older people, their relatives and carers. You can contact them by email at: advice@counselandcare.org.uk.

CHAPTER 4

PREPARING A BUSINESS PLAN

As a care home manager you may be asked to help to prepare the care home's business plan. In *How to write a business plan* (2001) Finch suggests that:

> *"You get one chance to make a good impression. Present a document that:*
>
> - *is persuasive*
> - *looks good*
> - *is free from spelling, grammatical or numerical errors*
> - *covers key areas*
> - *Contains the necessary supporting information.*
>
> *Having a sound proposal is great but first you must make a good impression and then you get the chance to demonstrate how good the proposal is."*

In his article *Application of business planning process in health care* in Nursing and Residential Care (2002) Makinson suggests:

> *"Plans need to address both long and short term goals. Plans should be linked to the aims, objectives and strategy of the organization."*

Care home managers must be able to describe clearly the services they are registered to deliver within the care home.

SWOT analysis

In *How to write a business plan* (2001) Finch describes the term SWOT analysis as simply

> *"Strengths, Weaknesses, Opportunities and Threats. This is shorthand for a system of business analysis that involves listing organisational ideas under each of these headings".*

Under the following headings are listed possible scenarios which may affect the care home.

Strengths

The care home manager needs to recognise the strength in the home. It may be the home's superb sea view location, first class bedrooms with excellent spacious en-suite facilities and nutritious but appetising food. Or it might be a home filled with a variety of social activities and stimulating trips to interesting places, arranged to cater for all tastes throughout the year.

The care home manager must be willing to promote the strengths, not only in the brochure, but also to every visitor who arrives at the front door of the home. The administrator or receptionist can be central in promoting the home's unique selling points. A simple, but most effective, tool is a clean and well-organised notice board. This should be up-to-date, relevant, informative and full of news items which are applicable to relatives and residents. A home newsletter can be an additional strength outlining the various activities and special atmosphere that is unique to the home.

Weaknesses (identified needs)

- The care home has been losing its competitive edge, it has a falling occupancy and social workers have stopped referring clients to the home.

- The atmosphere is changing from being relaxed to sensitive.
- A number of staff are leaving to work at a newly-built care home in the locality which is offering more money.
- The wages are poor, with carers only receiving the minimum wage.
- The care home has not been decorated for the last three years and looks tired. There is a smell of stale urine in some areas, including the lounge.
- The dining room furniture looks shabby.
- The kitchen is dirty and in need of a deep clean.
- The staff turnover may have left the care home without a natural leader and, as a result, the staff lack direction and they need to receive further training.
- Training may have been cut back dramatically due to the fall in occupancy and some of the staff are worried about the security of their jobs.
- There may not be a regular bus route to the care home and it appears that in the evening it is impossible to visit, unless the relatives have access to their own transport.

Opportunities

- The care home has recently been promised two clients from a local competitor that is closing down in the next three months.
- The care home has recently been upgraded, and a refurbishment has been authorised by the senior managers and owners of the home.
- The new brochure has been produced and is available for prospective clients.
- The staff have organised a summer fair and a local celebrity has agreed to open it.
- Advertising spare capacity in the local newspaper alongside the editorial about the summer fair means that the care home's profile is raised locally.

Threats

- The care home has lost clients to the new home that has recently opened down the road.
- The bus and train links are excellent to the new care home and the fees charged appear higher than the existing home.
- The care home is half-full and in need of a total refurbishment.
- The new care home manager has agreed to bring in some new staff and changes are designed to assist the staff in their development.
- It is clear that the staff have changed in their opinion about the home. They have, predictably, lost their original enthusiasm for it.
- Care homes without strong and effective leaders often go down hill very quickly.

It is vital that the owner and the newly-appointed care home manager agree on a time-scale for the changes they want to make. This agreement must be made at an early stage in the working relationship. It is essential that there is no ambiguity, as this can very quickly lead to friction and the break-up of any working relationship. Therefore minutes should be kept of any meetings held, and these should form the basis of any agreement.

In the end, you are aiming to present an action plan which contains realistic timescales and achievable goals. It should outline a recognisable pathway to get from the starting point to completion within an agreed timeframe. The secret of success is to design a robust action plan and agree a realistic budget. You should set targets for occupancy, wages to income, staff turnover and the control of sickness and absence.

Competitor analysis

Care homes can only survive if they have a clear understanding of what makes their competitors successful. There are many ways of discovering what is happening in other homes and intelligence comes from a variety of sources. Usually disgruntled staff are more than willing to tell managers what they are paid and what conditions are like, but remember the same type of information may be flowing out of the manager's home from their own staff. It is also important to note that it pays to keep commercial business information confidential: unscrupulous homeowners will be able to take advantage of a care home which has easily visible operating methods.

One of the key areas is setting the weekly fee, and the way these fees are negotiated with local authorities and private clients. It is essential to discover the key factors of influence and ensure that the relevant database is updated regularly.

Managers who are able to sell beds to prospective clients and their families can usually use these skills to provide services to local authority purchasers.

SETTING THE ANNUAL BUDGET

The company's finance department will be able to assist the new care home manager with the preparation of the care home's annual budget. In its simplest form, the budget with areas of proposed expenditure should be set out in one column against the income in another. The care home should only spend what it can afford and the most important aspect of the home is its staff.

It is important to take historical data into consideration, including the previous year's occupancy figures and the cost of payroll.

In the independent sector there are constant reminders of the cost of all items, and conscientious staff are also keen to develop more cost effective methods of delivering a high standard of care at the right price.

CHAPTER 5

IMPLEMENTING AN EFFECTIVE MARKETING ACTION PLAN

INTRODUCTION

All care home managers have a responsibility to their employers to maximise the potential of the home. They need to have a clear understanding of marketing and how it can be utilized to the best effect. The definition of the elements of marketing, known as the marketing mix, is:

The right product at the right price, promoted to the right people within agreed financial constraints, e.g. at a profit.

The right product

The type of service offered by the care home depends on the terms of the care home's registration. This registration dictates what type of residents can be taken into the care home.

Types of Resident who may be admitted to a care home
Residential
Low and High dependency
Nursing
Low. Medium High Nursing
24 hour continuing care
Elderly Mentally Infirm (EMI)
Young Disabled residents under 65 years of age
These are some of the categories of care

NB: If there is a variation to the agreed category of resident admitted to the care home an application must be submitted to the Care Standards Commission Inspectorate (CSCI). For example if you are asked to admit a person with Multiple Sclerosis for respite but she is only in her late fifties, then an application must be made prior to admission with the appropriate fee and a decision will be made by CSCI in due course. This process may take several weeks.

Market research will determine what specific care services are required in the local area. The Manager must identify local competitors and discover the reasons for their success, while aiming to improve their home's share of the market.

The right price

There is an on-going debate throughout the care industry concerning pricing of all care services, both in the public and the independent sector.

The true cost of nursing care will only be resolved when the criteria for such care are established and agreed by all parties. Hotel services in the home must also be costed accurately to achieve a realistic fee level.

In the future, detailed breakdowns of costs will be demanded by purchasers of care looking for the best value for money.

The right place

When individual residents and their families are choosing a place to live, they can be greatly influenced by its location and the community surrounding the care home. Other important considerations are the ease of access to local amenities and the availability of public transport routes for visitors who need to use them.

The appearance of the front of house is of paramount importance. The first impressions of the care home are found in the reception area. The gardens, buildings and car parking facilities are also key features which may ultimately attract potential clients to the care home.

Targeting promotion

Promotion of the care home can be achieved in a number of ways, for example through regular coverage in the local newspaper about interesting activities within the home. Professional staff dealing with telephone enquiries can also help to promote the home in a positive manner. Inviting potential clients to visit can stimulate their interest in the home.

Specialist brochures sent to a targeted number of people must outline the various services available. Any claims made by the home must be substantiated by clear evidence.

Social workers, GPs, ward sisters and charge nurses are often influential regarding any client and their family's choice of care home. Organising study days for local hospital staff may result in the care home being recommended for future clients.

Care home managers who say that they do not need to market their care home often fail to realise the importance of having a workable marketing strategy in place. They do not build relationships with potential purchasers of care, who then may decide to move their relatives to other competitors' homes.

Managers who do not recognise the importance of implementing a marketing action plan and fail to respond actively may witness a dramatic drop in occupancy and loss of the care home's good reputation.

Brand image

It is important to recognise the importance of branding, especially if the care home manager's home is part of a large care company. Today the brand may be as important as the service itself, as the general public may recognise the logo and strap line. Brands are so important that they are being regarded as having real value and are assessed as a tangible part of the assets of the company being sold or taken over.

If your care home is part of a premium brand, then this means it will usually appeal to people who want high-quality services and are prepared to pay for them. Remember that perception is everything. This applies in our every day lives. If you go to stay in London in one of the Hilton Hotels you expect a far higher standard of service than if you stay in a cheap bed and breakfast on the outskirts of the city. However you also expect to pay a premium tariff for the experience.

Financial constraints

The care home manager has overall control of the day-to-day costs of running the home and must therefore be aware of the revenue generated on a weekly basis.

DESIGNING A MARKETING ACTION PLAN

Designing a manager's action plan together will assist all staff to take ownership of their care home's marketing strategy. The following issues should be discussed at a staff meeting and actions taken to monitor and improve overall performance.

Telephone concerns

- Do you as the care home manager know how many enquiries are lost by the telephone not being answered either during or out of office hours?
- Do you often have difficulty getting through to your care home when phoning in out of hours or during office hours?
- Who is responsible for answering the majority of calls within your care home?
- Do you personally receive a monthly-itemised telephone bill?
- Do you check it and ask questions of others as to why the bill is so high?
- It may be possible to request the number of calls that remain unanswered.

Telephone enquiries

- Who is responsible for dealing with enquiries?
- Are the telephone enquirer's questions always answered in a standardised way?
- Is the enquiry form always completed with all relevant details, including contact telephone numbers, an accurate address and any further information?
- Have all staff received training in handling telephone enquiries? It is important for the care home manager to draft a short description of the care home so that any staff member can describe the location and size of the home and the facilities available. This information should be kept close to the main telephone in the care home and adjacent to enquiry forms.
- Staff must be reminded that they should always invite telephone enquirers to make a personal visit to the care home. It is advisable to set a time and date convenient to the caller and to make it clear that staff will fit in with whatever is most convenient for the client.

Sending the brochure

- The care home manager should devise a standardised letter which will be sent out with the brochure, information pack.
- Great efforts should be made to send the brochure and letter out on the same day that the enquiry is received. This can create a very favourable first impression.
- A copy of any of the care home's or company's newsletter should also be included in the information pack.
- The brochure should include up to date photographs of the care home including various views from the outside showing the building and gardens.

- The dining room, lounges and any special activities area or conservatory and one resident's bedroom and the hairdressing salon are always of interest to prospective residents and their families.
- It is useful to include a sample of the care homes weekly menu with various choices, a personal letter of welcome from the care home manager.
- A copy of a recent care home or corporate newsletter always adds the extra information illustrating what is happening here and now not five months ago.
- Remember to send all information with a typed address label and a standard sized envelope. Do not fold brochures and information as this does not look professional.
- Include a map and directions about how to find the home.
- Bus times and links are also useful if the relatives do not have access to a car. Also you may include the number of a local taxi firm to provide transport for the relative and prospective resident to view the care home.
- You may include a list of fees and include details of any extras that may be required to avoid upsetting relatives at a later date.
- Always check by telephone to ensure that the person has received the brochure, failure to check may result in the loss of a potential resident.

The prospective resident or relative's initial home visit

- First impressions of the care home are vitally important. The reception area front of house, the gardens and car parking facilities give any first time viewer a sense of what to expect.
- Is the care home well signposted? Does the sign outside the

care home look bright or old and dreary? If the latter is the case, then it should be changed quickly.

- Good signage is vital. If the sign is poorly positioned or too small, then any potential customers may drive past and go down the road to a competitor.
- Remember that a glossy brochure may seem deceptive, especially if the picture of the care home was taken in the summer and the home is being visited in mid-winter.
- Refuse bins should be in an enclosed area away from the entrance and must be kept free of litter.
- The staff should always appear welcoming and friendly and should wear their uniforms correctly.
- The visitors should always be encouraged to have a cup of tea or coffee in the manager's office before being given a tour of the care home.
- If the family is looking for ground floor accommodation and the manager only has limited vacancies, it is advisable to show the family to the area of their choice. If they are shown the entire care home they may feel it is too large.
- The manager should plan a route through the care home which is designed to show all visitors its unique selling points to their best advantage.
- The regional manager or sole owner of the home should check the enquiry folder on each visit to the home.
- The care home manager should analyse the number of enquiries and conversions. Clear reasons should be established for lost business and the database should be updated to show these. For example, a conversion may not be immediately possible if a client is waiting for funding from a local authority.
- All staff should be kept up-to-date with the strength of enquiries and the waiting list. The importance of maintaining an active interest in promotion of the care home and its reputation at all times should be emphasised.

- The home manager, senior staff or the care home's administrator should make the follow up telephone call within 12 hours of an informal visit.
- Many care homes fail to make follow-up calls and as a direct result a number of referrals are lost forever.
- All enquiries should be followed up by a telephone call within 12 hours of their visit to the care home.
- All enquirers who have been forwarded a brochure but have not contacted the care home should be followed up within three days.
- Any families who have not kept an agreed appointment must be followed up within 24 hours.

Monitoring enquiries

- Monitoring and accurate data collections are vital components of any enquiry system and must be checked by the care home manager on a weekly basis.
- The care home manager needs to analyse the number of enquiries per week. Conversions to placements will reveal clear details as to why people did or did not take up a place in the care home.
- Sometimes people may have to wait many weeks for funding of their placement.

The care home manager's role in marketing

- The care home manager's personality can make a massive difference to a home's reputation. Occupancy figures are often improved greatly by a highly motivated and charismatic leader, whose enthusiastic approach to marketing can turn a loss-making business into a very successful one.

- An introverted and reclusive manager is not usually associated with high occupancy levels unless there is a shortage of affordable beds in the locality.
- Office-bound managers often have problems recognising residents' names and if they show people around the home, this may be apparent to the visitors. The manager may not even be recognised by the residents and their families.
- A defensive care home manager can be seen as lacking enthusiasm and may seem moody.
- A care home manager who doesn't recognise the importance of keeping records of enquiries also fails to keep abreast of how well their competitors are doing. They cannot explain why the home's occupancy is falling.
- Some care home managers appear to reject the idea of marketing their home and some are resistant to follow-up enquiries.

Customer satisfaction

- Managers and staff need to be reminded that dissatisfied people do not recommend their care home to others.
- There are four main areas of concern to potential customers:

Housekeeping: cleanliness, smell and laundry.

Dignity: client presentation (clothes and personal hygiene).

Communication: keeping relatives informed about problems and progress.

Social care: organised activities. In the future there may be a national star rating system to enable people to compare care homes, based on a similar system to hotel star rating.

UNDERSTANDING PUBLIC RELATIONS AND USING THE MEDIA

Today care home managers operate in a very competitive market and any positive media interest is most welcome. Some larger care providers employ public relations (PR) experts who are retained to place stories in trade and professional journals on a regular basis.

The PR executive can manufacture a story, send out a press release, hire photographers and write captions, and even in some cases the accompanying story, in order to make the reporter's job easier. Presenting an article which is ready to print will almost guarantee its inclusion in the selected journal or newspaper. It is for these reasons that many trade magazines appear to run the same story almost word for word. The story and pictures originally came from the same PR source.

It is important to realise that employing PR people can have advantages, but they are also very expensive and must be able to justify their retainer. Larger companies may be able to afford their fees, but sole providers would find this additional expense prohibitive. However, it is useful to learn from their example and these can be seen as tricks of the trade

Photography

With the introduction of digital cameras it is now relatively easy to take pictures, download these onto a computer and immediately e-mail them to a newspaper. It is important to obtain written permission from any people who feature in a picture that may be published in a trade magazine or journal. The majority of people do not mind their picture being used, but others may see this as taking advantage of their status in the community for commercial means. This also applies if there are any celebrities who may visit the care home privately, as their agents often control their personal appearances.

A good story always benefits from being accompanied by a relevant photograph. A picture is worth a thousand words and must always be correctly captioned, interesting and in focus. Ideally it should possess a "Wow! Factor". Newspaper editors have access to hundreds of images every week, so make sure your photograph and story reach the top of the list and make it into the newspaper.

Press releases

The care home manager needs to involve the local press in covering any social activities in place to promote the home and must be able to attract the attention of the local newspaper editor. There is a tried and tested method of completing a press release. If this is followed, it usually results in at least getting a reporter or photographer to attend a function held at the home. Remember that there are several days to avoid. If the local newspaper is published on a Tuesday, then avoid holding your event on a Monday or Tuesday. These may prove to be the busiest days of the week. Therefore it is advisable to choose a day other than the weekend that does not clash with other events in the locality. There may be the opportunity to talk to a reporter on the telephone prior to setting a date for the event. Always include in any press release the following key points:

- Who is involved?
- Where is the event-taking place?
- Why is the event-taking place?
- When at what time and date?

An example of a press release:

Press Release
You are invited to attend
The Opening of the

Lakeview Care Home
Church Avenue,
Chapeltown,
Cumbria,
CH1 3TP
Tel: 01113 33444 Fax: 01113 33445

Mr Cliff Edge
Local author, mountaineer and filmmaker
On Friday April 13th 2007 at 11 am

The Lakeland Care Home will provide older people with dementia the warmth and companionship they need in a home designed to support local people and meet their requirements.

For further information please contact
Miss June Swain, home manager on 01113 33444

See the attached route map. Light refreshments will be available to members of the press in attendance.

Point of contact

It is important to establish one point of contact for the press from the care home, and this is usually the care home manager. The press appear to be a pleasure to work alongside when covering good news stories. However there may be a day when the press come to visit the home to follow up a newsworthy story and your relationship with them may seem somewhat different.

Many years ago I was the general manager of two large care homes in the North of England. At 3 am one morning I was woken by an urgent call from the night staff in a care home which was about 5 miles away. A ceiling had collapsed onto two of our residents. When I arrived at the care home the emergency services were in control. Fortunately both the residents were uninjured, apart from suffering from shock.

The following morning there was a number of reporters and photographers at the care home, all wanting quotes and pictures. The photographers wanted to take photos of the devastated room, but this access was denied and they had to be content with an outside shot. I knew I was fortunate that they were not more demanding. Members of the press are trained to get to the heart of a story and will try all kinds of tricks to get a scoop over their rivals.

The lesson that can be learned is clear: ensure that the care home has a "Dealing with the Press" policy. The following may be adapted to suit individual care homes.

A SUGGESTED PRESS POLICY DOCUMENT FOR CARE HOME STAFF

The Old Vicarage
Monkshampton Road,
Monkshampton,
Somerset.

Dealing with the Press policy

All staff please take note:
Staff must never speak to representatives of the press without the written permission of the care home manager/care home owner or, in the case of a corporate care home, the regional operations manager.

Members of the press are keen to get a follow-up story after an event which has taken place at the care home. They will try to gain entry into the care home, even posing as relatives. Staff must remain vigilant at all times and must refuse entry to those people they do not know or who cannot identify themselves. The Police may be called if the press representatives try and enter the care home without permission.

Photographers are under even greater pressure to accompany the reporter's story with an up-to-date photograph. Staff must direct the photographer to the care home manager. Remember to remain polite and that any comment you make may be used in the newspaper. It may be taken out of context and cause embarrassment not only to the staff but also to visitors to the care home.

Visitors may be approached for comments. They are free to talk to the press if they wish, but the easiest way to deal with any press enquiries is to issue a press statement via your Public Relations agency or your head office.

The press statement should include:

> The Old Vicarage,
> Monkshampton Road,
> Monkshampton,
> Somerset.
>
> **PRESS RELEASE**
>
> **FOR IMMEDIATE USE**
>
> Date: 26th July 2006
>
> **A brief outline of the incident:**
>
> A fire took place at 8pm in the laundry at the Old Vicarage, Monkshampton on Monday 24th July 2006. All twelve residents were evacuated from the care home to the local village hall by the staff on duty and fire brigade personnel in attendance. Two residents were kept in hospital overnight for observation as they had suffered from smoke inhalation. The rest of the residents were allowed back into the care home within two hours as the fire was brought under control.
>
> All relatives were notified immediately and the care home owner Mr John Jackson told the Monkshampton Advertiser
>
> **A quote from the owner if possible:**
>
> *"I am proud of the staff on duty and thank the fire brigade personnel who acted promptly in putting out the fire which could have had catastrophic consequences for the Old Vicarage. The extent of the damage will be determined in due course".*

NB: Never say how much damage has been caused as this could affect any future insurance claim. This should be left to the loss adjusters whose job it is to ascertain the cost of any damage.

"The two residents have returned to the Old Vicarage and are both recovering from their ordeal. The cause of the fire has not yet been determined."

ENDS:

Contact John Jackson on 07770998003 for any further information.

Find out how your staff reacted to an emergency when they were suddenly thrust into the limelight.

Lessons to be learned

- Care home managers should never assume that the press is on their side.
- Be acutely aware of the effect that negative publicity can have on a care home.
- It is important to foster good relationships with local newspaper editors.
- Staff should be debriefed by the care home manager after any incident involving the press. Dealing with reporters and photographers can be quite stressful, especially if the press stay around the care home for longer than a day. Remember that another local news story will come along soon, but it is hard to forget an incident in the care home that affects residents, relatives and staff.

Evaluating press coverage

The care home manager needs to be able to review media coverage by personally purchasing local newspapers and trade journals. Check the stories and advertisements competitors have had in the local papers recently. Why do you think the editor chose to run their story? Remember that editors are very busy people and they only have a limited number of pages to fill with news every week.

Reviewing newspapers allows care home managers to get a clearer understanding of the type of photographs and stories local editors want in order to inform their readers of the services and events happening in the local community. Some homes have targets of at least one story and photograph appearing in the local newspaper every month.

Keeping a record of press coverage

It is very useful to keep a record of press coverage in special albums which can be kept in reception. Often the best pictures are framed and kept on public show. Remember to date the press cuttings, and if residents are featured it is a nice gesture to give the relatives a framed print as a keepsake.

CHAPTER 6

DEVELOPING STANDARDS IN A CARE HOME

As a care home manager you may be faced with the prospect of setting standards. It is important to consult both service users and staff during the planning of any new standards. The purpose of setting standards is to ensure that there is a document available to all staff which can be used to measure their success or failure throughout the home.

There should be a simple process to follow to ensure compliance and this is measured through an internal and external audit process.

There are four key areas which you can initially develop:

- care standards
- environmental standards
- health and safety standards
- Management standards.

Care standards

When setting care standards it is useful to receive feedback from staff; residents and relatives on the present care services. Night staff should also be involved in any discussions about setting care standards. They are often overlooked in this process, but they do have a valuable contribution to make.

Achieving excellence in all care standards is crucial to the success of the care home, because it is in this area that residents and their relatives raise the majority of concerns and complaints.

There should be clear evidence that care plans are regularly evaluated and that clinical care reviews take place. This evidence will provide service users with confidence in the care home. Failure to record accurately these individual clinical reviews will lose the care home credibility.

A delegated senior member of staff should carry out a monthly care plan audit.

Care Plans need to be checked to make sure that the residents' needs have been identified and the necessary interventions have been carried out. It should also be shown that the care plans have been evaluated and updated as and when necessary.

Environmental standards

The first impression of the care home is the view from the roadside. Are the gardens clean and tidy? An overflowing dustbin gives the wrong impression of the care home and may discourage people.

All maintenance issues should be recorded in a book that must be monitored by the care home manager every week.

Fully qualified personnel must always be employed to carry out maintenance work on gas and electrical appliances.

Radiators should be covered and there should be nothing stored in the stairwells of the care home.

It is important to ensure that fire alarms and nurse call systems are maintained and checked regularly and all checks are recorded.

Health and safety standards

The care home manager is responsible for ensuring that the

health and safety of all residents, relatives, visitors and staff members is maintained at all times. Therefore it is necessary to form a health and safety group with health and safety representatives. Residents and relatives may raise issues that can be discussed by the representatives at the health and safety group's meeting.

There needs to be evidence of regular training in health and safety, fire safety, food hygiene and moving and handling, and all these sessions should be recorded in the staff's personal files.

Household chemicals need to be kept locked away and staff must be aware of the Control of Substances Hazardous to Health (COSHH) regulations.

The staff must remain diligent when working around the care home and follow the correct procedures when working with chemicals, knowing what action to take in the case of accidental spillages.

The head chef must be involved in the development of standards in the kitchen area. All foodstuffs should be stored in the correct place and at the correct temperature. Fridges and freezers should not be overstocked and their temperatures need to be accurately recorded. All foodstuffs entering the care home should be recorded. A daily record chart needs to be designed so that the care home manager can monitor it.

Hazards and infections

Care home managers will be expected to maintain a comprehensive list of potential hazard warning notices. They should be able to give advice on minimizing the risk of harm in their care home associated with using substances which may be harmful if used incorrectly. In the instance of the outbreak of any infections in the care home, the correct procedures must be put in place immediately to prevent further risk of the infection spreading and affecting other residents and staff.

See www.direct.gov.uk for further information regarding health and safety and environmental health matters.

Management standards

The care home manager is responsible for organising and holding regular staff meetings. The management standards should include a reference to budgetary control, ordering and utilisation of resources in the care home. There should be a schedule for staff training available in the care home. Customer care compliance should be monitored by the care home manager and all staff must be made aware of the feedback given by residents and relatives to ensure everyone is living up to residents' expectations. Marketing action plans need to be developed to ensure that all staff are committed to promoting the home.

Documentation and records

The exercise of developing standards in a care home can be daunting and it is vital to keep the process as simple as possible. When devising standards it is important to avoid the use of jargon. Before the documents are finally published, staff should be given the chance to discuss the various pieces of documentation in order to raise any issues. Remember, if members of staff have personal ownership, they are more likely to comply with individual components of the standards. It is difficult to provide discipline without the back-up of a clear set of guidelines, policies and procedures.

MONITORING CLINICAL STANDARDS

Implementing a recognised audit tool

The clinical audit process is a means of ensuring that clinical standards are monitored. The results need to be made public in an endeavour to improve the level of health care provision in each individual care home.

A recognised clinical audit tool is designed to quantify and provide quality feed back. If a care home fails to reach a score determined by the senior managers, it will be considered as a priority home and a team of specialists may be brought in to ensure that standards are raised to the parent company's recognised level of service provision.

Today the framework used as an audit tool is based on the Care Standards Act 2000 (Department of Health 2000). The sections are broken down into a point-scoring system and the audit tool must be designed to be used by an independent person. A baseline should be established against which an agreed set of standards can be measured, both quantitavely and qualitatively. Some large independent care companies have professional teams who are responsible for ensuring that all staff know what is expected of them and understand how they can implement the required standards within the care home setting.

Personal observation

One of the most effective ways of finding out how a care home is functioning and what the atmosphere is really like is to walk about and ask questions of all staff and clients.

Managers need to know how the domestic staff are feeling and should act upon their responses. In turn, the qualified staff have certain responsibilities to deliver high standards of care with the support of the manager and the rest of the staff.

Customer feedback

Customer surveys are important and the results should be analysed and acted upon by the manager. Sometimes staff can become concerned when they know that residents and relatives are being approached for their personal views on the services currently being provided. Customer care is vitally important and the staff need to recognise that customers' wishes are paramount. Staff in care homes should never take their clients for granted, because if they are not happy they may choose to be transferred to a competitor's care home.

Monitoring activities

One of the easiest and most effective ways of monitoring clients' social and leisure pursuits is to use a camera or camcorder to record events. These should be dated and displayed. Do not use old pictures and do not leave them on view for more than one month. The activities board should be updated weekly. However, it is very important that any resident's permission be obtained before photographs are displayed or put forward for any type of publication in journals or newspapers. Ideas for visits should come from the clients themselves, perhaps with some prompting from staff.

Promoting best practice

As the care industry becomes more competitive, there is a growing need to provide services which meet older people's expectations, and many older people now place social and recreational activities high on their list of priorities.

When searching for a care home designed to meet their expectations, clients and their families are committed to finding homes that will offer more than just a standard facility. The Department of Health (2001) emphasises that the routines of daily living and the activities offered in care homes should be flexible and varied to suit service users' expectations and personal preferences.

Care homes with one spacious lounge and a large television switched on from dawn till dusk are gradually being replaced by care homes which provide a number of smaller lounges designed to meet the individual needs of all clients. As people face retirement, we are meeting new categories of older person, for example those who have spent years on exotic foreign holidays, have been members of a gym and enjoy a keep fit culture. Many local councils run free swimming sessions for pensioners, so homes will be able to take advantage of this and other fitness activities which are provided with older people in mind. In their endeavours to produce quality care for older people, successful care homes now provide a range of social and recreational activities as standard practice. This will be discussed further under the heading of 'Activities organiser' on page 83.

CHAPTER 7

BUSINESS MANAGEMENT

KEY TO CULTURAL CHANGE

In *The new culture of therapeutic activity with older people* (2004) edited by T. Perrin, sound advice is offered to progressive care home managers wanting to overhaul the activity culture in their care homes. It is suggested that care home managers should develop the following attributes and facilities:

- be committed to person-centred care
- understand the value of activities
- be able to explain the value of activities to staff
- lead by example and show an interest in all events
- encourage all staff to be involved in activities
- give an activity organiser frequent, regular supervision
- commit to training and updating knowledge for activity staff
- include the value of activities within induction training
- establish the right environment for the residents
- provide adequate financial resources for functions, equipment and materials
- be committed to developing the potential that may arise from any situation or event
- accept that activity provision is about more than group sessions; that it involves one-to-one work as well as bringing the community into the care home.

Organisation

The care home manager must have the ability to organise all aspects of running a successful small business. It is vital to be able to see the big picture, and know what to do in a variety of situations without losing one's head. In a small group there are a number of factors that can make managers more effective in carrying out their duties.

Priority setting

A number of standard issues need to be addressed in care homes on a daily, weekly and monthly basis. These issues are as follows

- occupancy
- shift patterns and off duty
- contingency plans
- staff sickness and absence
- ordering provisions
- refuse collection
- wages to income
- clients' weekly fees
- staff recruitment and retention

Occupancy

The care home that is well occupied is, by definition, usually successful. Occupancy is of paramount importance. Staff need to be reassured that the occupancy remains high so that they know that the fees will pay for their personal wages, thus providing them with security.

In order to ensure that the care home remains viable as a business, it is important to establish target occupancy for each week of the year. It will be necessary to bear in mind that, as the occupancy increases, there is an expectation that the staff ratio will need to increase after consultation with the CSCI inspectorate.

Shift patterns and off duty

There are critical times in the year when staff shortages may be anticipated. These mainly occur in the winter and summer months and coincide with children's school holidays. The festive season presents unique difficulties. Managers who feel confident they have covered the off duty may find themselves in a dilemma around Christmas Eve when staff phone in sick and there is no cover. Nursing agencies are at a full stretch and the rates are so high that managers are left with no alternative but to cover the shift themselves.

While preparing staff rotas well in advance, it is advisable for the manager to ensure that staff have adequate transport arrangements made, particularly in rural areas where there may be a shortage of public transport. It is important that any staff who are finishing on the late shift are able to get home safely. Inevitably, taxi firms are prone to charge premium rates. However, forward-thinking managers check with staff and arrange lifts for people who do not have their own transport. In addition, public transport timetables should be displayed in the care home for the benefit of relatives and staff.

Contingency plans

It is important that managers devise written contingency plans which are available to all staff on duty. The Christmas and New Year periods can present many problems, not only with regard to staffing but also in case of any emergency. It is very useful to have a checklist in place with staff emergency numbers on display. Staff on duty will be reassured if they know in advance who to contact, such as the on-call pharmacy or GP. This information must be accurate. If it is not, a lot of critical time may be wasted. In turn, distress could be caused inadvertently to relatives and residents alike.

Determine what the staff's response would be in a variety of different scenarios. Ensure that staff are prepared for any emergencies that may occur, including fire and evacuation of the home. Is the home prepared to accept a number of residents from the local Social Services, should the need arise

The fire safety equipment must be checked in line with the care home's local policy but the following good practice must be in place. Fire extinguishers must be checked by the manufacturers at least annually. The fire panel must be checked at least once a week and a record made of the date and time this took place. Fire drills should be held monthly during night duty as well as during the day. Contractors should check the smoke alarms every three months.

Staff sickness and absence

Contingency plans regarding staff sickness are important, and any absences should be reviewed carefully following the event. Agency staff should only be used as a last resort, as the premium rates can have a massive impact in the end-of-month analysis. Nothing should be left to chance and it is important to remember that adverse weather conditions can often occur unexpectedly. Care home managers have a responsibility to monitor staff sickness and absence, as care homes cannot afford to pay salaries to staff indefinitely. The manager needs to act in a sensitive manner, as prolonged ill health can sometimes have a devastating effect on a person's standard of living.

Ordering provisions

The normal procedure for the ordering of provisions is that the care home should have enough stock for two weeks. At the festive season a little extra provision always comes in useful. Remember there is often limited freezer space, and fresh produce should be ordered as close to Christmas day as possible. Similarly, if possible, fresh foodstuffs should be ordered for delivery on New Year's Eve.

Residents' menus should reflect the festive season, but special dietary needs and vegetarian alternatives must be available, as usual.

Nutritional supplements and foodstuffs must be ordered and delivered in sufficient quantity to cover this holiday period.

Refuse collection

The removal of any waste is extremely important. It is the responsibility of the care home manager to ensure they know when the local council is due to collect the care home's waste. In addition, they should know when private contractors will be removing clinical and domestic waste from the care home. The care home manager should ensure that extra storage containers are ordered if there is to be an extended time between collections. Disposable bags must not be stored outside the special containers, as the bags can be ripped open by vermin.

Wages to income

Any care home needs to be able to survive profitably. One of the most important financial indicators of a good business is the wages to income percentage. In simple terms if a care home is 100% full with 20 beds at all times and enjoys a waiting list, this means that with fees at £500 per week this will give a total income of £10,000 per week. The wages bill is £5,000 per week, therefore the wages to income percentage is 50%.

Clients' weekly fees

Perhaps one of the most challenging and demanding aspects of the care home manager's role is having responsibility for the fee structure alongside the owners of the care home. Maximum fee levels are essential if care homes are to survive in the competitive market place. Many care home managers find it difficult to mix care with finances, and to this end they prefer not to be involved in the annual fee negotiation round. Those senior managers involved in setting fee levels often devise a formula which reflects national trends on fees.

Staff recruitment and retention

Implementing a staff recruitment and retention policy will result in a stable work force which is valued and able to provide continuity of care for clients.

Staff recruitment can be made easier by inserting a professional advertisement in the press, followed up by a simple-to-follow job description and a neat, easy-to-complete application form. Remember to short-list potential staff carefully, looking for experience and a good staff mix of mature staff and those who have less experience.

Staff will only stay in the post if they feel valued financially. They also need to feel supported by training so that they can deliver care in a systematic and creative way. Care homes which do not adapt to the changing demands of clients and purchasers soon empty and close rapidly. In the next decade there will probably be a dramatic reduction in the number of places providing care. The present government's interest appears to lie in the development of domiciliary care, and the future of large institutional-type care homes may in time be phased out forever. Therefore it is important to retain staff who can be flexible in the work place and deliver care in a variety of settings. Homes may need to diversify into home support teams to ensure that their own staff remain in employment. Care homes that fail to adapt to these changes will inevitably have to close their doors forever.

TIME MANAGEMENT

We are all vitally affected by the way in which we manage time. Every individual needs to be disciplined in their approach to managing their time efficiently. Care home managers can become more effective in producing better outcomes in their daily work routine.

Some people thrive on meeting deadlines. For example, newspaper journalists who have to meet deadlines every day produce interesting stories which are read by thousands of people over breakfast the next day. The simple skills we need to manage other people are exactly the same ones that we require in order to manage ourselves.

Good managers must be able to plan and ensure that the plan is carried out, not for half the time, but all the time. Plans often come unstuck when people forget a plan or try and go off on their own and devise a new plan.

In *Organise Yourself* (2000) Caunt suggests that in order to implement a method of planning and tracking your time you need to be able to:

> *"Determine your objectives, break assignments down into their component tasks and identify what you will need from others in order that you can complete your own tasks".*

It is important that you keep a close check on your meetings and appointments and on your contacts. Planning your day in the care home is important because staff need to know when you have important deadlines to meet. Sometimes you may arrive at work with good intentions and a crisis happens which can send your plans out of the window. Some people make a habit of finding excuses not to deal with the important priorities.

Planning care

Planning care and managing the care home's resources have equal importance and cannot be treated as individual components.

Individualised care plans are essential to provide staff with clear guidelines to deliver a model of care. This will be effective and easily monitored and will provide clients with the chance to make informed choices about the type of care they receive while in the care home.

A partnership must be formed between the client, family and staff to ensure that everyone's expectations are met to the best ability of the staff team under the leadership of the manager.

Delegation

Delegation of tasks allows care home managers to concentrate their skills on high priority issues. This gives other staff the opportunity to carry out other important tasks, for example the ordering of stock and ensuring that the laundry and housekeeping services are working effectively.

Valued senior staff will provide the care home manager with the type of support required to ensure a good working relationship. To delegate a task does not mean that care home managers are walking away from their responsibilities.

In my personal experience, good care home managers also return to check on the work carried out by junior staff, they never assume that something has been done. If the person who was given the job to do on the manager's behalf fails, then ultimately it is the manager who has to accept the responsibility.

Activities organiser

Care homes which have appointed an activities organiser to implement a structured activities programme are generally able to demonstrate greater co-operation between staff and residents. There are still many care homes in this country that sadly treat residents' activities in an *ad hoc* manner without consulting either individuals or their relatives. Social and recreational activities planned in consultation with the care home's residents and their families are often very successful. Large independent care companies are now investing heavily in DVDs, videos and even plasma screen televisions, allowing older people to watch up-to-date DVDs and videos rather than just terrestrial television.

Today's exciting activities may range from holidays and day trips to parties and different kinds of entertainment in the care home, eg. concerts featuring local musicians or sing-along entertainers. On a more permanent basis, the care home manager and the activities organiser can set up groups that concentrate on appreciation of the arts, writing, poetry, physical exercise, musical appreciation, bridge and chess. A good home will have a library that is well stocked, not only with books but also with CDs and videos which can be borrowed by individual residents.

In the future a computer room may be provided for the residents' use. This could include a printer and digital cameras and might be used for recording special events throughout the care home.

Supporting evidence

It is very useful and desirable to keep an up-to-date record of events that have taken place. These can be stored in photograph albums illustrating client and staff outings, entertainment, group work, and social parties, and can be used as documentation to show prospective clients. Only the best photographs should be used as a record of any event or facility. It is advisable to display a variety of photographs covering a number of events, rather than lots of photographs covering only a few events.

Residents' individual views

To provide support that allows residents to maximise their individual potential, it is essential that managers, staff, volunteers and visitors listen to the older persons' own views and wishes. Their comments about social activities should be included in the care home's local monthly newsletter. Promoting events through the newsletter is also useful for keeping everyone up-to-date with what is happening regularly in the care home.

Staff may discover positive results in the way clients approach a more active lifestyle. For example, clients who are encouraged to take a more active interest in life outside the care home appear to have raised awareness of their personal dress, hygiene and self-esteem.

Community links

The Department of Health (2000) states that residents should be able to maintain regular contact with their family and friends within the local community. The home manager has a responsibility for ensuring that members of staff are trained to appreciate the importance of social interaction between clients and the local community. Links should be made between the home and local community groups, such as local churches, mosques and synagogues, recreational centres and shopping centres. One major supermarket recently offered to sponsor a coach to take clients from a local care home to a destination of their choice, which proves that business relationships can make a real difference to clients' every-day lives.

STAFF TRAINING AND DEVELOPMENT

Training needs analysis

Newly appointed care home managers should be able to ascertain what training staffs require. They need to consider:

- the types of training which have already been delivered
- when and by whom the specific training was delivered
- how many staff have achieved NVQ and at what level

In addition, every staff member needs to have an individual discussion with the manager to establish what training they need and what training they have already undertaken. This will establish a starting point from which the manager can provide a training programme.

Staff supervision

Staff are entitled to support from the care home manager, and supervision allows staff the opportunity for individual discussions about any issues which may concern them. Supervision must be carried out at least six times per year (Department of Health 2000).

Staff appraisals

It is very important that all staff receive positive feedback. Care home managers are responsible for developing clear objectives for each member of staff and should agree an action plan and a timescale in order to achieve their individual personal goals.

The member of staff should be given at least a fortnight's notice in which to prepare for the appraisal meeting. The care home manager in turn needs to prepare and to ensure that the right amount of time is set aside. The meeting should be held in a quiet environment, without interruption from telephones or other staff.

If the manager has practised a continuous appraisal technique, then there should be no surprises in store for the member of staff. Discussing any member of staff's strengths and weaknesses must be done objectively, but managers should stress that there is always room for improvement.

Criticism should be constructive. Managers may decide to examine the member of staff's job description in greater detail. The purpose of any appraisal is to motivate and provide staff with the prospect of better pay and perhaps promotion.

Public speaking and training sessions

Care home managers are committed to staff development, and as part of that undertaking they are required to provide in-house training themselves.

It is important that people expected to speak in public not only possess the relevant knowledge, but they should also be able to deliver an interesting, factual and thought-provoking message. The care home manager should be confident and motivated to carry out this task. The effectiveness of any training session can be measured by the amount of information recalled by participants.

Preparation is essential if you are to feel confident about your presentation. It is vital to check any electrical appliances such as slide projectors, video recorders and PowerPoint presentations, before people enter the room. There is nothing worse for a group of staff than having to sit and wait while the person talking to them struggles with the technology.

Teaching methods

During a two-hour training session it is advisable to use a variety of teaching methods. You may want to split the group into two or three sub- groups in order to get people talking to each other. Each sub-group needs to appoint a spokesperson to feed back to the whole group.

Video

Sometimes you may be told about a training video, but you should always check its relevance and suitability for the group. Never rely on anyone else's word that a training video is relevant, because if they are wrong it could be very embarrassing for you. If you decide to use a video as part of your presentation make sure you can illustrate some examples that apply to the care home. The interactive use of video will ensure that staff are involved in discussions about real life issues with which they can identify personally.

Timing

Remember to leave time for questions and answers from the staff group when planning your training session. Do not allow yourself to be side- tracked as this will waste everyone's time and can lead you to overrun your allocated time.

If you are not an experienced public speaker there is a possibility that you will try and rush through the presentation. It is therefore recommended that you practise the delivery of the presentation beforehand. This will give you the opportunity to add more information or remove some to make sure you stay on schedule.

Conquering nerves

Often very experienced public speakers suffer from nerves before giving important presentations. Some people may feel physically sick, and this can only be overcome by trying to relax. Remember to focus positively on all the aspects of your talk.

- You have researched and planned your presentation.
- You have practised and got the timings just right.
- You are among your own staff who are keen to learn.

Tips for public speaking

- Speak clearly and slowly.
- Avoid repetition.
- Do not just read your notes; try to make eye contact with members of the group.
- Do not talk with your back to the group.
- Remember that you know the beginning, middle and end of your presentation. You are in control.
- If you do not know the answer to any question, admit it and say you will find out the necessary information.

Summary

The art of public speaking takes years to master. It is useful to take note of people who speak regularly at major conferences. Really successful conference speakers can forego visual aids and, by speaking passionately, still enthral their audiences. Remember that by sharing your knowledge you will inspire staff to follow your example. Ultimately, the residents are the main beneficiaries of a well-informed staff.

CHAPTER 8

REFURBISHMENT OF A CARE HOME

Perhaps one of the most interesting and challenging aspects of the care home manager's role is being involved in a major home's refurbishment programme.

The overall planning of any such refurbishment programme should be undertaken with the full cooperation of the owner, the manager and staff.

Large companies employ their own teams of interior specialists who will plan and help the manager to agree a final scheme that will be fully costed. It is essential that residents and their families are made aware of the proposed programme well in advance and are informed of any inconvenience that may take place during the refurbishment.

PLANS

It is vitally important that any plans drawn up and agreed by the company be discussed in the first instance with the manager. Refurbishment may cause some disruption, be it noise levels or the inconvenience of having a lounge or dining area out of use for a few days.

Plans should be agreed and act as the guidelines to any refurbishment programme. In the past, people have offered to undertake small refurbishment programmes without adequate planning and preparation. This can result in loss of business and overspending on the agreed budget. It is vital that the timetable for work should not be allowed to slip, as a number of people can suffer as a direct consequence.

FURNITURE AND FITTINGS

All chairs should be covered in a fabric which can be regularly cleaned and retains a modern, comfortable appearance. All furniture must be fire- retardant and meet recognised British safety standards. Always check that the furniture has an appropriate fire safety label before placing any orders with suppliers.

Be certain to check delivery times with suppliers, as furniture may be delivered in flat packs and need assembly on site. Chairs usually take between six to eight weeks' delivery time. Managers should be aware of the legislative and servicing requirements to comply with the care home's insurance policy.

Floor coverings

Carpets and flooring must be professionally fitted and all floor coverings should be designed for industrial rather than domestic use. It is essential to seek expert advice. Although this may mean spending more money initially, in the long term it is well worth it.

Decorations

It is important to get professional advice when it comes to redecorating a care home. This redecoration programme should not be compared with decorating a private house, as there are a number of factors which need to be born in mind. Consideration needs to be given to the residents' needs as well as to the impression a new colour scheme would give.

The reception area and corridors are the showpieces, because first impressions are so important. Getting quotes from decorators is not easy, because inevitability there are unseen extras. For example, there may be refurbishment work to do before the redecoration itself can be carried out.

Sometimes clients are given the opportunity to help choose the colour schemes in their bedrooms. There are thousands of colour schemes and wallpaper books to wade through, and the professional decorator can offer practical advice based upon years of experience.

Dining room

Tables need to be large enough to accommodate wheelchairs, yet small enough to appear homely rather than clinical and institutionalised. Dining room chairs may have arms and should be fitted with skids to enable movement without danger to client or members of staff. The manager should check the desired specification in the brochures. It is preferable to install a wood laminate floor as this is much easier to keep clean and tidy.

Pictures: artwork and photographs

Whenever there is a refurbishment project it is reasonable to purchase new pictures for all areas of the care home. There are specialist artists' outlets which can offer framed modern prints at reasonable prices. Pictures help to brighten up the home. Individual residents' choice is important when choosing pictures in the public areas such as corridors and the residents' public lounges.

Types of Beds

The type of beds purchased for the clients can vary in price. The variable-height beds are expensive but are preferred by staff. When purchasing beds, it is important to remember that hoists are now used routinely and as a result it is necessary to provide beds which allow hoists to be used in the bedrooms. Cheap furniture can easily get damaged and often needs replacing much earlier than furniture which is perhaps more expensive but will last longer.

CHAPTER 9

SURVIVING REDUNDANCY

INTRODUCTION

Senior managers who have spent many years working in the care industry may at some time face redundancy or have their position terminated.

Redundancy can happen to anyone, no matter how experienced they are or what position they hold in the company. Any planned changes of ownership, mergers of care companies or the appointment of new senior personnel may result in certain staff being earmarked for a move within the company or being made redundant.

It is important to accept at the outset that it is the post being made redundant, not the person. For instance, due to downsizing the post may amalgamate with another post. It is vitally important that if you are chosen for redundancy you quickly find out the notice period and the offer and financial settlement to which you are entitled. You will also need to find out what is to happen to your pension. Can it be transferred to your new employer? It is often advisable to seek legal advice through the Citizens Advice Bureau (CAB). You can find them in your local telephone directory or go to www.adviceguide.org.uk or www.citizensadvice.org.uk. In order to save time, it is advisable to ring for an appointment before going to visit the CAB.

The starting point is to discuss the redundancy with your immediate family. The first feelings are usually anger and shock, which may manifest themselves as bitterness and personal resentment against the company's senior management and fellow employees. People often say "Why me?" and proceed to accept the future without any thought of where their next post will be. In order to overcome this malaise, the best plan of action is to be pro-active and determined to use the situation to your advantage.

CV and covering letter

The plan should begin with an up-to-date CV, as discussed on page 2. Your CV is vital in order to create a good impression. It should be no longer than two well-spaced A4 pages and should contain basic information about you and your career to date. This should be succinct, honest and factual, designed to persuade people into calling you in for an interview. It is a good opportunity to sit down and reflect on all the skills you do possess.

A covering letter to accompany the CV should be written to any leading company, but this may not necessarily be as a response to an advertisement. Many senior management posts are never advertised nationally, but instead leading care providers may employ a company of head hunters in an endeavour to find talented people throughout the care industry.

Looking for work

Newspapers are good places to start looking for jobs, as are nursing professional journals. Many jobs are never advertised and usually a small group of people known as head hunters search the country for successful managers. This is not a quick fix and head hunters can only match companies with tried and successful candidates. They are recruitment specialists who are trained and employed on a contractual basis to identify and introduce outstandingly talented people to potential employers. You may be approached by a head hunter if they are alerted to your skills, reputation, and experience in the care industry. If you are approached, then you should listen to what the head hunter can offer you on behalf of potential employers. However, you must remember that the head hunter will speak to a number of high-calibre candidates. They cannot guarantee success, but they can improve your chances of getting to the final selection process.

If you cannot find a head hunter or you are not approached, then it is important to find a post yourself. Once you have a list of possible jobs, send for application forms. It is important to keep a record of any posts applied for and the closing dates for returning application forms.

The secret of success is to be persistent. Interviews can be very demanding and you must be confident in your approach to each post. It is very important to learn as much as you can about the company to which you are applying. Sometimes you may have to choose a post that you do not feel confident in undertaking, but remember that often a change of direction in your career can be a very good thing and a new start can be very productive.

One way of finding out about available posts is to write an introductory letter to a number of large companies to see if there are any vacancies to match your qualities and qualifications. Your letter may just be kept on file, or you may be invited for an interview and be successful in gaining a post with a prestigious company. If you are on a head hunter's target list you may be introduced to a number of different companies. Using head hunters has the advantage that they will be keen to match you up to a suitable position, so you won't waste time going after inappropriate posts.

It is vital for your family to be supportive in your quest to get a new job. It is worth remembering that sacrifices may have to be made in order to achieve full-time employment.

Recruitment consultants charge introduction fees but cannot guarantee success in the challenge to find new employment. They do, however, keep your CV on a database and will not charge you for this service. The agency will act as a go between for you and any potential employer.

They have years of experience and provide excellent communication links.

Your new employer pays them a percentage of your salary as an introductory fee.

If you are a qualified nurse or an experienced care support worker, then you may wish to sign up with a nursing care agency. Also remember the old fashioned job centre. This has now been revitalised by the government, ensuring that all jobs are now computerised and available on the internet.

Many people now search the internet for job vacancies and can also receive information regarding positions by email. Some newspapers, such as The Guardian, offer to match your CV with any vacancies and alert you by email if suitable vacancies arise.

References

Employers' references are very important, so before leaving the post from which you have been made redundant, think towards future prospects.

Interviews

Refer to the section starting on page 3 to remind yourself about interview techniques. Prior to interview read through the job description and the personal specification for the post for which you have applied. What are the prospective employers looking for in their appointment of a new manager or senior regional manager?

The outcome of any selection process is not pre-determined, therefore everyone short-listed has an opportunity to secure the post, dependent upon their performance.

Personal finance

It is important to sort out your financial affairs. Inform your bank and any creditors that you have been given a redundancy notice as soon as possible. The earlier you let them know, the easier it is for them to offer you appropriate support. *Do not cancel* any overdraft facilities you may have in place, as these can be difficult to re-instate. Demonstrate the fact that you are looking for work and this will give the bank manager confidence that you are able to achieve your ambitions.

You may be fortunate and receive a lump sum as part of your redundancy settlement. This may be invested or go some way to paying off your mortgage or other debts. It is important to seek professional advice rather than trying to deal with the matter on your own.

The realities of redundancy

Never be over-confident, because if you fail to achieve your goal then it is harder to manage. However, if you really want to achieve in management you have to accept that it is not an easy option and there are always many people wanting each available post. Management posts are not for the faint-hearted. The price of success can affect family life and there are many sacrifices you may have to make to achieve full-time employment. It is vital for your family to be supportive in your quest to get a new job.

Redundancy can happen to anyone, no matter how experienced they are or what position they hold. The country as a whole often faces periods of recession in various industries and many people are made redundant. The news of redundancies may make the local newspaper and sometimes reach local television news programmes. Sadly, the problems continue long after the newspapers have been thrown away and the stories forgotten.

Care homes may have to downsize due to falling occupancy and high staff turnover. Because of the threat of closure many care homes are choosing to sell to large companies. A change of ownership may bring with it changes of use or diversification, and this may lead to staff having to be made redundant. Anyone facing redundancy is legally entitled to personal notification by his or her employer. As previously discussed, people who face redundancy may have initial feelings of anger and frustration with a degree of bitterness towards their employers. There is a genuine feeling of disbelief.

Often, those who have been made redundant feel that they have failed their colleagues and families. Many relationships suffer, sometimes irreparably, due to redundancy. Occasionally people who are facing redundancy keep it a secret from their families, hoping that they can find a job before the redundancy notice is finalised. There are occasions when a business has to make staff redundant, but subsequently there is an increase in occupancy so that the redundancy notice is lifted.

People have been known to pretend to carry on going to work even though they have lost their job. Keeping the fact that you have been made redundant a secret is not at all advisable. It increases the burden and deprives you of the support which you need. It is important to be positive about finding alternative employment as soon as you feel you are able to do so.

Make a document file and store all your details, including all job contacts, advertisements, useful addresses and any copies of letters written to prospective employers. The secret of successful job hunting is to be organized and enthusiastic, and not to give up. You must realise that you will often not get the first job for which you apply. You have to find your unique selling point. What can you do for the new company? What are you major achievements? Why are you looking to join a new company? Find out as much as you can about your prospective employers. Find out who the key players are, go online and find out as much as you can about the company profile. How many beds and staff do they have? The internet will provide detailed information which can help you to gain an advantage over other candidates.

Meticulous filing is important. When you receive a letter inviting you to interview, attach to it copies of the original advertisement, letter and application form you have submitted. At this point it is important to ask your current employer for permission to use their name for reference purposes.

Relocation is always an option and may be necessary in order to gain worthwhile employment. Relocation expenses may be available for the right candidate. Remember that if you choose to move to another country you need to be aware of the unique legislation concerning the provision of health care.

A combination of self-belief, enthusiasm and the desire to attend a number of interviews will ultimately help you find a new post. Being positive is very important and you need to maintain faith in your own abilities.

Negative feelings are perfectly normal especially if redundancy hits you when you are over 40 years of age. Ageism does sadly still exist in the workplace, but it is possible to overcome prejudices. While you are unemployed you may be made to feel like a second-class citizen. You may even become depressed and require medical support from your GP. However, the simplest way to resolve this is to whole-heartedly devote your efforts to the job-seeking process.

There are many people who, faced with redundancy, choose to emigrate and find work in another country. There are others who decide for personal reasons to change career direction. While there is not much demand for redundant health care managers, there will always be a need for the bedside nurse and care workers. Therefore, if you have a nursing qualification or experience and skills in care, then you should be able to find employment.

You may be at a time in your life when reducing your hours or taking on a job with less responsibility will come as a relief. Remember that, as the children leave home, you may be left with spare time. You don't need as much money because they have gone through University and even one of them has left home altogether. If the mortgage is paid then you may be in a position to sell your house and move to somewhere smaller and release the capital to have that well deserved Caribbean cruise you'd always promised yourself.

Redundancy need not be the ultimate failure but can be seen as the golden opportunity to find a new lease of life. Many people work at the same place for so long that they become part of the furniture and moving on is never an option. However, once redundancy is suggested then the nurse or carer may see this as the chance to make a fresh start. Treating the threat of redundancy in positive manner may bring rich rewards. Not only financial, but in meeting new people and starting out on a new and exciting journey. We are never too old to learn new skills and it is perhaps the only opportunity you will have to try something new, fresh and challenging.

THE MANAGER'S VIEWPOINT

Perhaps one of the most devastating pieces of news you can receive is that you have been made redundant. The bitter pill can be sweetened with the reassuring words "remember it's not the person but the post that is being made redundant". The news is never easy to impart. As the care home manager, it is important to ensure that the news is broken in a face-to-face interview, and always in private.

Passing on bad news can be made easier if the person is provided with an honest reason for their forthcoming departure from the company. Redundancy can often be a cloud that has a silver lining, and moving from a small company to a new challenge should act as an incentive to those people who find themselves at this low point in their careers. Once the news has been given, it is important to allow staff to devise a plan for finding themselves a new position.

- The member of staff should update their CV, ensuring that all information is accurate and succinct.
- They should reflect on the type of post they would like to apply for, bearing in mind that it is not a foregone conclusion that the first post applied for will achieve success.
- There are many well-qualified people looking for every post that is advertised, either locally or nationally, so the key is to apply for a position about which one feels confident. It is important to ensure the personal profile and qualifications match the requirements of the new company.
- The person facing redundancy should be given adequate and reasonable time to attend interviews and search for jobs.
- There is a chance that people feel angry, bitter and resentful and there is sometimes a case to be made for

people to be sent on paid leave so that they do not come into work. This may avoid potential disruption in the workplace.

- Managers who are released from their jobs are often left bewildered and after visiting the job centre find they are very low in mood.

As an employer, it may be helpful if you consider the following aspects with an employee you have had to make redundant.

- They may not sleep and may be faced with the stress of not only having to find new employment but the possibility of losing their home. In some extreme cases they are at risk of losing their families.
- It is essential to be honest with potential employers and tell them clearly what has happened. This approach will pay dividends and will ensure there are no surprises from previous employers, who may not wish to provide a good reference for their own specific reasons.
- It is important for family and friends to rally round and support at these difficult times. Some friends may be able to supply positions within their own companies and surrounding areas.
- Being jobless is very much like parenthood. You cannot have empathy with people who find themselves in the position until you have experienced those feelings yourself.
- Never take work for granted, because it is one of the most rewarding experiences you will ever have. To be without work is almost like a bereavement in the family.
- Employers need to be mindful of the consequences of their actions. If people are failing in their role then we must be in a position to offer support and guidance.
- Managers need to be streetwise and recognise and embrace the need for change. Experience and being nice are no

longer enough to survive in what has become, in parts, a cut throat business.

- Profit is important in order for any care home to survive and prosper, but we must retain a sense of fairness in all our business activities which complement our vision and values.

CHAPTER 10

THE WAY FORWARD

The satisfaction and pleasure of becoming a successful care home manager is to be tempered with some words of caution to the newly-appointed person. The way forward is to take staff team members with you on the journey. Responding to the challenges of change and inspection in the care market means that only the fittest and most highly-motivated care managers will survive.

Today it appears to me that throughout the United Kingdom there is an exclusive club developing for a number of high-stake companies. Takeovers and merges will ensure that just a few major players dominate the independent care sector Therefore, if you wish to carve out a career in care management, you must be aware of the future career pathway that is open to you. It would be advisable to gain a business qualification such as an MBA which would give you the theoretical background to assist in your management career.

The next step up from the home manager is the area manager, and then next position is that of the regional manager. After several years, you may aspire to become an operations director and you may one day become the managing director of a large company.

In order to achieve your ambition in life, you need to be able to realise your dreams and aspirations. You can and will be a successful care home manager, but first you must believe in yourself and your abilities.

I am currently working as an independent care management consultant and I have been responsible for undertaking a number of interesting and challenging projects for major care providers.

Throughout my working day I am constantly reminded of the importance of the care home manager in ensuring that the residents receive the highest quality care and support.

In addition to care home managers' clinical responsibilities, they have the overall responsibility for running a successful business.

The care home manager is like a football coach, teaching theory and leading the team by example. The staff in turn deliver care and support which is recognised and appreciated by everyone associated with the care home.

Remember a good reputation takes years to develop but minutes to lose and you are only as good as your last admission into the care home.

Always try and finish your working day by. asking yourself one question,

> *"What have I done today that makes me feel proud?"*

Try and achieve a work/life balance which takes your family into account. There is always a danger that they may take second place to your role as care home manager. Take time off to recharge your batteries. Give other team members responsibility through delegating certain tasks.

To end on a positive note, you have one of the most rewarding jobs in care today and your future is in your own hands.

Be passionate about care and you will find that people will be motivated to go the extra mile. Never ask others to do what you are not prepared to do yourself. The results you achieve will surprise even you.

Good luck in your future management career, it is a long journey but well worth it in the end.

REFERENCES

Ashurst A (2005) We should value overseas nurses. *Nursing and Residential Care* **7(10):** 443

Caunt J (2000) *Organise Yourself.* Kogan Page Ltd. London.

Chambers N (2003) The diverse role of the care home manager. *Nursing and Residential Care.* **5(7):** 342–334

Chambers N (2003) What kind of leaders do we need in our care homes? *Nursing and Residential Care* **5(8):** 389–391

Clutterbuck D (1994) *The Power of Empowerment.* Kogan Page Ltd, London.

Department of Health (2000) *Care Standards Act.*

Finch B (2001) *How to write a Business Plan.* Kogan Page Ltd. London.

Forsyth P (2002) *How to Motivate People.* Kogan Page Ltd. London.

Greenwood D (1999) *The Job Hunter's Handbook.* Kogan Page Ltd. London.

Harvey-Jones J (1989) *Making it Happen – Reflections on Leadership.* Fontana/Collins, Glasgow.

Johnson G, Scholes K (1993) *Exploring Corporate Strategy.* Prentice Hall, London.

Makinson G (2002) Application of business planning processes in health care. *Nursing and Residential Care* **4(4):** 185–187

Mannering K (2000) *Managing Difficult People.* How to Books Ltd. Oxford.

Penhale B and Manthorpe J (2001) Sexuality and residential care: issues for staff and clients. *Nursing and Residential Care* **3(6):** 252-253

Perrin T (ed) (2004) *The new Culture of Therapeutic Activity with Older People*. Quay Books. London.

Sewell P (2001) Career Management with a Curriculum Vitae. *Nursing and Residential Care* **3(10):** 468 - 469

FURTHER READING

Ashurst A (2002) *Positive Customer Care – an aide memoir.* Quay Books, Dinton.

Braham J (1997) *Benchmarking for People Managers.* Institute of Personnel and Development, London.

Caunt J (2000) *Organise Yourself.* Kogan Page Ltd, London.

Coleman V (1988) *Stress Management techniques.* Mercury Books. London.

Drucker P.F (1963) *The Practice of Management.* Mercury Books, London.

Finch B (2001) *How to Write a Business Plan.* Kogan Page Ltd, London.

Forsyth P (1999) *30 Minutes to Write a Report.* Kogan Page Ltd, London.

Forsyth P (2000) *How to Motivate People.* Kogan Page Ltd, London.

Forsyth P (2001) *Developing Your Staff.* Kogan Page Ltd, London.

Ghaye T and Lillyman S (2000) *Reflection: Principles and Practice for Healthcare Professionals.* Quay Books, Dinton.

Gibson F (1998) *Reminiscence and Recall.* Age Concern, England.

Greenwood D (1999) *The Job Hunter's Handbook.* Kogan Page Ltd, London.

Kennedy G (1986) *Everything is Negotiable.* Arrow Books, London.

Mannering K (2000) *Managing Difficult People.* How to Books Ltd, Oxford.

Nash S and Nash D (2002) *Deliver Outstanding Customer Service.* How to Books Ltd, Oxford.

Page S (1995) *Introductory Marketing.* Stanley Thornes Ltd, London.

Young A (1987) *The Manager's Handbook.* Sphere Books Ltd, London.

USEFUL WEBSITES

All websites were active in July 2006.

Citizens' Advice Bureau
www.adviceguide.org.uk or www.citizensadvice.org.uk

Commission for Social care Inspection (CSCI)
www.csci.org.uk

Counsel and Care
www.counselandcare.org.uk

Department of Health
www.dh.gov.uk

Health and Safety Executive
www.hse.gov.uk

Internurse
www.internurse.com

Registered Nursing Home Association
www.rnha.co.uk

Royal College of Nursing
www.rcn.org.uk

See www.direct.gov.uk for further information regarding health and safety and environmental health matters.